About The Authors

Dr Gillespie received her MD and urologic training from the University of California at Los Angeles, and she practices in Beverly Hills. Her lectures on cystitis and urologic problems have won her international attention professionally.

Medical writer Sandra Blakeslee writes for *The New York Times* and other major publications.

YOU DON'T HAVE TO LIVE WITH CYSTITIS

How to Avoid It – What To Do About It

Larrian Gillespie, MD

with

Sandra Blakeslee

CENTURY

LONDON MELBOURNE AUCKLAND JOHANNESBURG

First published in Great Britain in 1988 by
Century Hutchinson Ltd
Brookmount House, 62–65 Chandos Place, Covent Garden
London WC2N 4NW

Century Hutchinson Australia (Pty) Ltd
PO Box 496, 16–22 Church Street, Hawthorn, Victoria 3122, Australia

Century Hutchinson New Zealand Ltd
PO Box 40–086, Glenfield, Auckland 10, New Zealand

Century Hutchinson South Africa (Pty) Ltd
PO Box 337, Bergvlei, 2012 South Africa

Printed and bound in Great Britain by
Anchor Brendon Ltd, Tiptree, Essex

British Library Cataloguing in Publication data

Gillespie, Larrian
  You don't have to live with cystitis
  1. Women. Bladder. Cystitis
  I. Title   II. Blakeslee, Sandra
  616 6′ 23

  ISBN 0–7126–2394–9

Designed by Jacques Chazaud
Illustrations by Richard Paschal

To all the women
who dared to seek a better way
and
to our families

Contents

Acknowledgments

I would like to express my appreciation to Mr. Richard Turner-Warwick and his wife, Dr. Margaret Turner-Warwick, for "adopting" me into their family.

LARRIAN GILLESPIE, M.D.

The names and circumstances of clients in case
histories have been changed to protect their privacy,
except for Pamela Sue Martin.

What This Book Will Reveal to You

Cystitis: Free at Last!

If you accept the widely held attitude that women are fated to develop bladder infections, this book is not for you. If you think that cystitis, as such infections are called, is "no big deal," you should stop reading now. But if you reject this widely held idea, we can start to build a partnership in dealing with the problem.

This book emphatically challenges the belief that cystitis is as inevitable as the occasional menstrual cramp. As a surgeon specializing in disorders of the urinary tract, I have found that cystitis is preventable. It is not some kind of primeval female curse that we all must endure. Rather, it is an abnormal bladder condition that is more often than not caused by some functional (rather than anatomic) problem. Using common sense, its causes can be found and treated. *You don't have to live with cystitis!*

Your grandmother, however, was perhaps less fortunate. A hundred years ago, antibiotics (used so effectively today to kill bacteria in the bladder) were not known. Yet women developed cystitis then for many of the same reasons that they develop it today. In this book, you will learn what is both new and old about cystitis.

Over the centuries, numerous cures and palliatives were devised to treat the symptoms of cystitis. These remedies, many of which were excellent, have been passed down to us today. I will tell you why some work and others do not, which ones are valuable, and which ones lack merit. You will also, I hope, have your eyes opened about the many old wives' tales that purport to explain the causes of cystitis. For example, women are told they get bladder infections from sitting on the cold ground, from having too much sex, or from having too little sex. Such beliefs, which are total nonsense, have persisted because no factual information has ever been offered women to supplant those old wives' tales.

Probably no one has ever explained to you the many ways cystitis can develop, why it can recur, and how easy it is to prevent. This book will give you that information step by step. It is an attempt to bring women from the Dark Ages regarding cystitis into the Age of Enlightenment. It should help you discover why you are getting bladder infections or why the symptoms of cystitis won't go away. It lays out fundamental principles that you can use in getting to the cause of your problem. It tells you how to maintain your urologic health.

You Don't Have to Live with Cystitis

One of my major interests in recent years has been figuring out the many causes of cystitis. Contrary to what you, your mother, your grandmother, and all your family's doctors have been taught for generations, *cystitis is curable*. The prevailing notion that you are fated to develop a painful bladder infection at least once during your lifetime simply is not true. The fact that you may have already developed repeated infections is heartbreaking.

I have treated thousands of women for cystitis. Most infections could have been avoided had my patients known a few simple facts about female anatomy and how bladder infections arise. Indeed, cystitis is now an ailment most women can avoid. Urologists are learning more each day about the intricate mechanisms of bladder function and how the urinary tract works. New biochemical findings about this system are leading to better treatments and prevention of disease.

Tragically, American women continue to make more then 8.9 million visits a year to the doctor's office because of cystitis. It is the most common affliction prompting women to seek medical attention!

I am constantly surprised by how little my patients know about their urinary tracts and by the way they perpetuate myths about cystitis. But the patients are not entirely to blame.

To this day, urologists are taught that women may never be cured of cystitis. Women get cystitis again and again, we are told, because women are "built funny."

You should never get a bladder infection unless there is some anatomic or functional reason underlying the disorder. But if you are like most cystitis sufferers, your anatomy is perfectly normal. Your infection can be traced to a functional cause—that is, it is something you can easily prevent if armed with common sense knowledge.

Common Sense Urology

The medical specialty of urology appealed to me for several reasons. I love puzzle solving, and urology is a field with few hard and fast answers. There is no single formula for any single disease that makes everyone well. The urologic system is particularly complicated, and many parts of it can go awry in an infinite number of ways. Every patient is unique and needs to be assessed individually.

Working with patients has taught me how to be a keen observer. My medical school preceptor and I used to play a game. As we went on rounds, he would suddenly point to a patient and say, "What is wrong with that one?" I had to focus immediately on anything I could pick up about the subject at hand. It was like the game we played as children in which we looked at a picture for fifteen seconds, looked away, and then wrote down everything we could remember about it. Medicine is similar. You observe each person and focus on what he or she is saying. Today, I can often figure out what is bothering a patient just by looking at the way she sits, walks, or holds her body.

Throughout my residency training at UCLA, I was always the "but" person; I'd say, "But . . . what about this observation? But . . . what the book says doesn't make sense. But . . . this can't be right." When things didn't work, I wanted to know why not. I wondered aloud if something might be wrong with the logic being applied. Have we reached only part of the answer? Should we be content with "This is the way it is?"

It was this unwillingness to accept edicts, as passed down in some medical textbooks and by some professors, that led me to put more trust in my innate common sense on matters of female urologic function and health than in all those edicts.

Everything you will read in this book is based on my practice of urology for the past six years. The information does not necessarily reflect the opinions and training of the UCLA urology residency program or those of the American Urological Association or other urologists. Rather, this book distills for women my own distinct approach to urology.

As a urologist, I treat men, women, and children. A few years ago one male colleague told me, "I always knew it would take a woman to figure out women's problems. Put a woman into urology and things will change."

Women in Urology: A Splash in the Pan?

As the first woman ever to be accepted into UCLA's urology program, I did not realize it was unusual for a woman to choose this specialty. I presumed, in my naiveté, that women were involved in all fields of medicine. It was only upon applying for a residency position that I was informed by other (male) urologists that no woman, to their knowledge, had ever been trained in urology in the entire United States!

As it turned out, this was not true. Currently there are seventy-four women urologists in this country, but many of our male colleagues are surprised to find out that we exist. Comparatively, we Americans are progressive: Finland boasts only one female urologist; the United Kingdom and Yugoslavia each have only a few; and most of the other countries in the world, sad to say, do not offer a single accredited female urologist. There are fewer than 100 women urologists in the world—an average of one for every 400 million people.

I chose urology because I believed a woman could offer special insights into this fascinating field of medicine that affects so many other women. After all, at least half of all urologists' patients are women.

A few years ago, I presented a paper, "Women in Urology: A Splash in the Pan," about the history of women in the field.

Everyone laughed at me, saying the talk would last but two minutes. Instead, I could hardly contain my lecture within the allotted twenty minutes.

Although over the centuries very few women have practiced urology, it turns out that one of the earliest specialists was a woman. Her name was Trotula, and she practiced in Salerno, Italy, during the eleventh century. Historians tell us she was a very attractive, feminine woman who treated both male and female patients. Her prescriptions for urinary tract infections and stone disease were numerous. Her teachings include twenty-nine observations she made on urine and she is credited with the first description of the skin manifestations of the disease we now call syphilis.

During the late tenth century in Egypt, the demand for women in urology was great. Kidney stone disease was very common, yet male physicians were not allowed to touch women. Abou'l-Quâsim, a noted surgeon in the court of the Caliph of Cordova, stated that "one must find a woman well versed in urology but they were few and far between."

One of my colleagues recently noted that "overwhelmingly, the gynecological literature of medieval Europe was written for a male medical audience and was a product of the way men understood women's bodies, functions, illnesses, needs and desires."

It seems that for hundreds of years, right up to the late 1800s, when the industrial revolution brought women back into professional roles, women urologists were virtually nonexistent. It was a struggle for women back at the turn of the century to become recognized as full-fledged surgeons with medical degrees hung neatly on the wall. Many male medical school professors believed that women did not require and were not fit to receive the scientific education needed to become a first-rate physician. As one professor said, "For their own sake, it is not desirable that they should pursue some of the studies necessary such as anatomy." It was thought that the study of natural science would injure a woman's character. In the medical schools of those days, male students were assigned a dissecting laboratory separate from the female, or "hen," medics. Women were not allowed to dissect male genitalia. Instead they were given a castrated papier-mâché model of the male body.

But some women rebelled. Sophia Jexs-Blake, founder of the Royal Free Hospital for Women's Education in London, stated at the turn of the century, "If a woman's womanliness is not deep enough in her nature to bear the brunt of any needful education, it is not worth guarding."

I found a trail of many women who had practiced urology, some of whom developed innovative surgical and medical treatments. Unfortunately, none survived in the field. They were forced to treat only women and children or to turn to gynecology. The work they did was credited, as was then customary, to their male mentors.

In recent decades, many excellent women physicians fared no better in attaining what they really wanted out of medicine. Virginia Apgar, who developed the Apgar scale used worldwide to assess the health status of newborn infants, always wanted to be a surgeon. Yet her male colleagues told her that she did not stand a chance. She regretted to her death that she allowed them to talk her out of a surgical career.

By the early 1970s, when I was receiving my medical training, myriad social factors had changed, for the better, a woman's chances of entering surgery, urology, or other specialties formerly practiced almost exclusively by men.

Women have been allowed into these fields and are beginning to make unique contributions to the practice and study of medicine. Women urologists, I daresay, are beginning to make a difference in how diseases of the female urinary tract are viewed and treated.

When you think about it, the way the medical community divided up female anatomy long ago made no sense. The gynecologists got the reproductive tract and the urologists got the urinary tract (except for bladder hernias, which only gynecologists were then taught how to repair). As a result, when a woman feels burning when she urinates, caused by a vaginal infection, she is punted to the gynecologist. When she feels burning when she urinates, caused by a bladder infection, she is turfed back to the urologist. This is the famous punt and turf game of specialized medicine.

As medical consumers, women are beginning to ask that the

rules of the game be changed. Why not have specialists trained in what might be called *urogynecology?* The female reproductive and urinary tracts—like those of men—are intimately connected. Physicians who treat women ought to understand the complexities of both systems. But today this is simply not the case.

Grasshoppers and Ants

Private practitioners do not, as a rule, conduct basic research. But when confronted with a fundamental paucity of understanding about women's urologic health, it becomes necessary to investigate these problems scientifically. As a result, I have published numerous original articles about cystitis and other urologic problems that tend to affect women. Much of this book is based on those scientific inquiries and results.

Someone once told me that scientific inquiry is conducted by two types of researchers, grasshoppers and ants. The grasshoppers are the mavericks, the bold leapers, the ones who ever propose new, possible answers to tough questions. The ants are the establishment, the detail gatherers, the phalanx of workers who ultimately follow many of the insights made by grasshoppers. Both ants and grasshoppers are necessary for the advancement of science.

But if I had a choice, I would be like the grasshopper. Not all the leaps win gold medals. But they do stimulate awareness of medical issues and help promote research into long ignored women's problems. Some of my leaps may prove wrong and some will prove right. Some treatments and therapies I use today may seem crude in twenty years, but if they stimulate scientific thinking in the right direction, they are worthwhile. Forward progress is extremely important and I feel I have contributions to make.

The work I do is ongoing. As you'll see in this book, at no time do I claim that we completely understand each problem and here is the exact answer to each question. Rather, you will see that we are following simple logic in analyzing each question. We look at how problems evolve and how individuals can have many interconnected factors that lead to their cystitis, incontinence, or other urologic health problem.

The book is not meant to take the place of an office visit with your doctor. It is not a substitute for medical care. Rather, it is a guide to help you achieve a better working relationship with your own physician through knowledge.

I suspect that as you read the book, you may be struck at how simple and obvious some of the discoveries appear to be. I can hear you saying, "Of course! Why didn't they think of that ages ago?" But the solution to many of these puzzles about cystitis, incontinence, and other problems appear simpler than they really are. They remind me, to use a show business analogy, of Fred Astaire's dancing. He made his performances look simple. Yet his motion picture frames were timed to the second. It was hard work that gave the illusion of simplicity. It is hard work, too, that is leading to a new understanding of female urologic health.

You Have Common Sense Too

I tell patients to use their common sense with regard to bladder infections. Women are intelligent. If something makes sense, it must have some basis in being correct. But if you can't understand a treatment or technique and it doesn't make sense to you, it can't be the right approach to your problem. For example, a woman given antibiotics for a bladder infection when none exists might ask, "Why am I taking these pills?" The answer, "To prevent you from getting an infection," doesn't make a lot of sense. The faulty logic of this common practice—some women are routinely given antibiotics to prevent bladder infections when they have no infections—is immediately apparent to anyone who thinks about it. But if you are intimidated by physicians and you want to get better, you don't necessarily think logically.

This book will teach you how to work with your physicians so you get the best value for your medical dollars. You want to understand what is being done to your body. If it doesn't make sense, you might be seeing the wrong physician. Don't be afraid to keep changing physicians. Find the one who can help you unravel your mystery. This book may help serve as your validation—that you are right to keep looking for answers to your problem—until you find that practitioner.

When you go to a new physician, you may find little opportunity to ask the kinds of questions that would help you figure out why you are getting cystitis or having other problems. Being in private practice, I sympathize with how little time most physicians have. With the demands of surgeries, emergencies with patients, and difficult diagnostic problems, we find ourselves hurrying through each day with never enough office hours.

On the other hand, I firmly believe that patients should spend far more time with their doctors. They should be equal partners in diagnosing and treating any medical problem. Of course, the only way to establish such a relationship is for the physician to spend more time with each patient. Patients need to be given more information about their bodies, reasons for problems, why treatments are tried, and what to expect from any course of action.

Time is precious in a healing situation. Knowledge is imperative. This book is an attempt to combine the two and help you regain and maintain your health. When you understand what is happening to your body, you can tackle any problem with far greater strength.

By educating yourself, you will also be helping your doctor. Urology is a fast moving field. Physicians who left school twenty years ago may not, for example, have been exposed to some of the latest information about cystitis. Please understand that because medicine is so vast an enterprise, and none of us can be an expert in everything, most doctors choose to specialize in one small area; thus we tend, as physicians, to choose an area of personal interest.

Why You and Not Me?

When I began private practice, I became uncomfortable not knowing what caused cystitis in my patients. I didn't like giving medication without knowing why the patient got the infection in the first place and how we could stop it from happening again.

I am a healthy, sexually active woman. Yet I have never had a problem with my urinary tract. I have never had a bladder infection. As women continually seek my help for urinary tract infections and other problems, I always ask myself, "Why? Why is she different from me?" By asking this basic question, I have been able to shed light on several aspects of disease affecting women's lower urinary tracts.

No one, for example, had scientifically studied the effect of birth control methods, particularly the diaphragm, on cystitis. No one, for example, had stressed to patients the close link between lower back problems and cystitis. *Yet the bladder is one of the most sensitive indicators of lower back problems,* and many women with recurrent urinary tract infections can trace their problems to simple but nagging lower back injuries. In addition, a fundamental misunderstanding of female anatomy led thousands of women into having unnecessary surgery of the urinary tract.

And then there is the guilt. Many patients tell me that they feel it is all their fault they are having urinary problems. After all, if they hadn't had too much sex, they wouldn't have an infection. Some tell me that they are terrified to have sex, fearing they are doomed to repeated infections. Some have told me that they think a bladder infection is the way they have to "pay" for an emotionally satisfying experience.

Most women go to their gynecologists for treatment of their first and second urinary tract infections. But when you have had three or more bouts, you may be referred to a urologist to find out why you have the problem.

As many women came to see me with the symptoms of cystitis, I became unsettled on learning that many had rarely had their urine cultured. It was assumed they had bacterial infections of the bladder and they were prescribed antibiotics over the telephone. This practice, as I discuss in Chapter Two, may lead to a chronic disease called interstitial cystitis. It is, in my opinion, the orphan disease of women.

I have developed several approaches for treating interstitial cystitis based on strategies to stabilize cell membranes, and these are discussed in Chapter Three. While much basic scientific research is involved—and all the answers are not in—you should be able to understand the nature of this disease and how various environmental factors give rise to it.

I also discuss the effects of interstitial cystitis on sexual function and on mental health. Strategies for coping with chronic pain and stress have been developed by my psychologist patients who have this disease.

In Chapter Four you will find guidelines on how to be a patient. In my experience, women are often unprepared for their doctor's appointment and speak from emotion rather than from an orientation to the facts. If you have a chronic health problem, you do not want to be dismissed as "another hysterical female" by doctor after doctor. By preparing for your next visit to a physician, you can overcome that bias.

The next chapter, Five, walks you further through the anatomy and function of each component of the female urinary tract. I detail why women are urologically different from men and may help you better understand your body. It tells you why your urethra cannot be in the "wrong place"—that is, too high or too low—thus causing urinary tract infection.

In the beginning of my practice, I did what I had been trained to do in medical school. I would look first for an anatomic explanation for your problem. This stems from the still widely held belief that female bladder function is affected by our "peculiar" female anatomy—that the urethra is "too close" to the anus and "too short" to keep bacteria out of the bladder. The perineum, the skin bridge between the anus and the vagina, is said to be a "breeding ground" for bacteria that get into the bladder.

Let me assure you, there is nothing wrong with the design of the female perineum! The perineum wouldn't have survived the trial of human evolution if it were such a handicap. The female urethra is not a shortened, amputated version of the male urethra but a separate, integrated unit with different functions. Therefore, other factors must be involved in the causes of cystitis.

After finding most of my patients to be anatomically normal, I began to suspect that what I had been taught about anatomy and cystitis in residency didn't answer all the questions. It became a very frustrating experience for both me and my patients to have them undergo expensive, invasive tests only to find no good reasons for their infections.

Indeed, anatomic abnormalities are rarely discovered in mature women; such abnormalities almost always show up in childhood. Fortunately, pediatric care in the United States is so excellent that very few children with anatomic problems are missed. They reach adulthood without chronic urinary tract infections.

Some women have their urethras repeatedly dilated—that is, forced open with instruments—to prevent further infections. But what has been done to try to stop cystitis in women is based on the same male understanding of female urinary anatomy and function. This practice of dilation does little to prevent infections and harms the patient. It is what some urologists call "the rape of the female urethra."

Chapter Six is devoted to urinary incontinence, a rarely discussed topic. Yet some 12 million Americans suffer from incontinence—that is, they leak urine! You will learn about the different kinds of incontinence and how to treat each one. For example, a treatment available for one type of incontinence can be done in my office. You walk in wet and you walk out dry. Also, there are simple exercises that you can learn to reduce the symptoms of incontinence.

In the next chapter, Seven, I discuss women's urologic problems that arise during menopause. Three out of every five postmenopausal women in the United States have had a hysterectomy, and over 700,000 hysterectomies were performed on women of all ages in 1983 alone. This operation can have profound effects on a woman's urinary tract. In seeking to relieve lower pelvic pain, many well-intentioned gynecologists have performed hysterectomies, only to find that the operation did not correct the problem and take away the pain. So that unnecessary hysterectomies will not be done, I believe gynecologists and urologists need to join together in a common field such as urogynecology.

Hormone replacement therapy is a very controversial subject that can also have profound effects on a woman's urinary system. You need to understand the trade-offs involved in such therapies to maintain a healthy bladder.

Chapter Eight delves into the effects of pregnancy on the urinary tract. For example, many women void differently when pregnant and some are misdiagnosed as having bacteria in their urine. Thus, they may be put on antibiotics even though they are perfectly healthy. You can avoid this problem through a simple technique that I will describe.

Chapter Nine is about children. After explaining some common anatomic problems, I describe my theory of what causes bed-wetting and how to stop it. A concept described in Chapter Two—the leaky cell membrane phenomenon—applies to bed-wetting. I'll show you how diet and a simple medical treatment can stop bed-wetting and give children control over their bladders.

Chapter Ten discusses bladder cancer, giving you an idea of what treatments are available. I believe patient attitude toward this disease is an important factor in treatment. You will learn how to deal with the emotional stress of cancer and how to look at trade-offs involved in different treatments.

Finally, Chapter Eleven discusses how nutrition affects the way cells function in your urinary tract and reveals dietary guidelines that improve the symptoms of interstitial cystitis, bed-wetting, migraines, and colitis. You will learn how to protect your bladder through a wise choice of foods and vitamin supplements.

The Appendixes include information on the Interstitial Cystitis Foundation, a national source for up-to-date findings on this disease; a guide to the medications most commonly prescribed for urologic problems and what medications should be avoided by interstitial cystitis patients; and a description of the tests and procedures used by urologists.

Throughout this book, you will read the stories of my patients and how they were helped. Every story is true, based on real people with real problems. To protect their privacy, only first names have been used, with one exception: Actress Pamela Sue Martin, who is the honorary chairwoman of the Interstitial Cystitis Foundation, asked that her name be used to draw national awareness to this disease and its treatment.

My Goals

This book has several goals.

First, I want to give you knowledge because with knowledge comes power, in this case the power to stay well.

Second, I want to help you learn how to be a successful health care client. As women, we often have great difficulty relating facts to our physicians unless we are secure in that relationship. My goal is to give you the confidence to know that you can share personal observations with your doctor and not be accused of making emotional, irrelevant remarks. At the same time, I want you to learn how to take responsibility for your own health. Patients who get better do so through tremendous personal effort, or as one woman recently said, "I think that each of us has within the power to heal." I take this to mean that you are responsible for your own wellness and road to recovery.

Third, I want to teach you about your body. It has become very clear to me from my own office practice that as a first step to permanent well-being, most women need to know more about how their urogenital system really works. As a rule, a woman who comes to my office for the first time does not know where her urethra really is located. Men get that knowledge simply because they can look at each other.

Another of my goals is to better understand the cellular physiology of disease. On the level of molecules and cells, what factors contribute to problems of the female urogenital tract?

This book will give you the answers to this and many other basic questions about your urinary system's health. And it will help you find out why you are getting cystitis and how to avoid having it ever again.

ONE

Why You Have Cystitis

A ny woman who has had cystitis cringes from the viewpoint, held by many doctors, that three or four bladder infections a year is no big deal. The pain of these episodic infections is excruciating. For hours and perhaps days, she can think of nothing else as her bladder controls her life. And while these common bacterial infections are not life-threatening, they are temporarily life-shattering. Cystitis won't kill you, but it does make life miserable.

Cystitis can occur at any time in males and females of any age. Children, grandmothers, husbands, and sisters can develop it, for various reasons. It is most common, however, in sexually active women. So to begin explaining how bladder infections develop in healthy people, we'll start with Tricia's story.

It was Monday morning. Tricia woke up and stretched, remembering the delightful evening before. It had started with a dinner date and wonderful conversation and ended with Tricia in the arms of her favorite man.

But now, as she sipped a first cup of coffee before work, she noticed something was not right. She had a strange need to urinate. There was a tingling sensation in her urethra and a feeling of pressure in her lower abdomen.

She had the feeling that she needed to go to the bathroom and needed to go now. First, while on the toilet, she removed her diaphragm. It had been in place about eight hours now, and she felt assured that it had worked correctly.

Moments later, Tricia's feeling of well-being was shattered. When she urinated, it hurt horribly. There was a searing, burning sensation as warm urine trickled out of her bladder. It felt as if someone were pouring acid on an open wound. She squeezed out everything she could and went back into the other room.

She thought, "What am I going to do?" At work, she had a report to finish before a 2:00 P.M. committee meeting and at least a dozen telephone calls to make. This felt like a bladder infection coming on. She knew from experience that it could knock her out of action for several days. She gulped down three glasses of water and went to work.

At the office, Tricia's symptoms grew worse. When she went to the bathroom, she noticed her urine was a smoky color. Later, there was a bit of blood on the tissue.

A colleague gave her cranberry juice and a vitamin C tablet. Another told her to wash her vagina with copious amounts of cool water. But Tricia developed a gnawing pain around her pubic bone and it seemed every time she urinated, the pain was more intense.

By 4:00 P.M., Tricia was in agony. She desperately wanted medical help. All the water, cranberry juice, and vitamin C had not helped. She couldn't stand the discomfort any longer. What went wrong? Why did this happen now?

Cystitis and Your Anatomy

Women who develop bladder infections constantly ask these questions. Why me? Why now? To understand what went wrong, you need to understand how your urinary tract is supposed to work and to know which parts of your body are affected by cystitis. (For more details on the anatomy and function of the urinary tract, see Chapter Five.)

Amazingly, most women do not know where their urethra is located. Many of my patients are embarrassed to tell me they

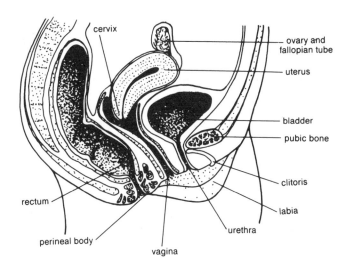

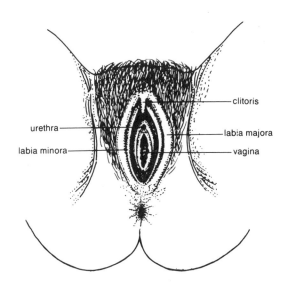

Figures 1-1, 1-2, Anatomy of the Female Pelvis

don't know this simple fact. Others think they know where the urethra is located but are way off track.

Look at the illustrations on page 17 of the female lower urinary tract. Notice that the urethra is located just above the opening of the vagina. In fact, the vagina and urethra share a common tissue plane. The urethra is a specialized tube that connects the bladder to the outside. It transports urine out of the bladder.

Your bladder is located in the lower part of your pelvis, in front of your uterus. It is very much like a collapsible balloon in that it expands as it fills and contracts as it empties. It stretches slowly to make a reservoir for the urine that your kidneys are constantly making.

The female urinary tract is highly efficient and—this is a very important point to remember—it is designed to perform differently from the male urinary tract. Many physicians, even urologists, mistakenly believe that the male and female urinary tracts

---

Frequency, Burning, Pressure

When bacteria multiply in your bladder, they cause you to feel sensations of burning, pressure, and frequency. Each symptom is correlated with how bacteria affect the tissue that lines your bladder.

The bacteria actually adhere to your bladder lining by secreting an enzyme called *urease*. They then split the urea in urine, which results in the production of ammonium salts and produces that burning sensation and special urine odor. As the protective lining is weakened by bacteria, urine crosses over to the cells and tiny capillaries that make up the bladder wall.

When urine comes into contact with these cells, it stimulates special chemical receptors that make you feel the need to urinate. These receptors are overly and improperly stimulated by the urine, giving rise to the sensation of frequency. Some women with cystitis may feel the need to urinate as often as every ten minutes.

When urine gains access to the nerves that lie between cells lining the bladder, the nerves fire. Smooth muscle within the bladder contracts, giving you the feeling of pressure.

are anatomically equivalent and that the female urinary tract is a shortened version of the male urinary tract. This is not so. The female urinary tract serves very different functions and women have different urologic problems from men.

When women void, the urethra is placed so that urine streams down over the labia, the vagina, the perineum (the skin bridge between the vagina and rectum), and then exits over the anal sphincter. We are built like French bidets; we thoroughly cleanse ourselves as we urinate. Any bacteria adhering to surrounding tissues is continually washed away. The next time you urinate, pay attention to how this works. Notice how the urine washes you off.

However, if something prevents the bladder from emptying efficiently, bacteria can be left behind—either in the bladder or on surrounding tissue, where they may find an ideal environment in which to multiply and thrive.

It is clear that one bladder infection means that things are not working according to nature's design. *Something*—and there are many possibilities—is compromising your natural system.

Let's Get Rid of the Old Wives' Tales About Bladder Infections

Before exploring the causes of cystitis, I want you to carefully consider five basic concepts that should dispel some of the misinformation or myths that you may think are true. These are common sense concepts that will help you understand why you have contracted one or many bladder infections.

• *Bacteria often get into the bladder during sexual intercourse.* This is natural, normal, and nothing to worry about. The urethra is next to the vagina. During foreplay, bacteria that thrive on the perineum are easily mixed with vaginal fluids and massaged into the urethra by your partner's fingers. During the repeated thrusting motion of intercourse, the bacteria may work their way into the bladder. This truly is nothing unusual or threatening. It is normal!

• *The bacteria are your own.* They can come from your perineum, vagina, or anus. They *do not* come from your partner. In other words, he is not infecting you with his germs.

• *Your body has natural cleansing mechanisms.* Most of us don't get bladder infections because bacteria are washed away when we urinate after intercourse. Urine cleanses the bladder, the bladder neck, the urethra, and the vaginal area as well. Moreover, the bladder lining has intrinsic bacterial defenses in its tissue. Even when bacteria stay in there for several hours after intercourse, infections don't normally occur.

In 1961 doctors demonstrated this fact by placing stool directly into the bladders of medical students. After the students urinated a few times, the stool and the bacteria it carried were completely washed away. There were no infections. (This study was very critical to our understanding of cystitis, but it also gives you an idea of the regard doctors have for medical students.)

• *A urinary tract infection is not a problem of bacteria getting into the bladder.* It is a problem of bacteria *not* getting *out*. This is a mechanical or functional issue. When what goes in cannot get out, that is a setup of conditions for an infection to occur.

• *There is more than one way for bacteria to get trapped.* One is that something is obstructing your normal flow rate. A second is a neurologic problem, such as damage to the nerves in your lower back which are associated with bladder function. In such cases, there is residual urine in the bladder which can feed the growth of bacteria. This leaves you susceptible to a bacterial infection.

Always Get a Urine Culture

If, like Tricia, you wake up one morning with what you think might be a bladder infection, you need to do one thing right away: get a urine culture done. Many things can cause the symptoms of cystitis, and you *do not* want to take antibiotics if you do not have a bacterial infection.

After work, Tricia went to a nearby walk-in health clinic and left a urine sample. As her urine was "cooking"—left in a warm place overnight so that any bacteria present would colonize and show up the next day growing on the culture dish—Tricia began a course of treatment to knock out what we were pretty sure was a bacterial bladder infection. At this point neither she nor I knew what had caused her infection, but her discomfort was so great that we decided to treat her while awaiting results of the urine culture.

How to Give a Urine Sample

When you give a urine sample, the nurse will give you a sterile container and ask you to catch urine in midstream. Lean way forward so urine does not have a chance to flow up into the vaginal opening and back out again (this happens easily if you lean back against the toilet seat). Be sure the urine does not come in contact with any pubic hair. Your goal is to catch a bit of urine that has come directly from the bladder and is not contaminated with any bacteria that might be residing outside the bladder. Urinate for a moment, to wash away bacteria around the urethral opening, and then place the cup under your stream of urine. If you do not have a bladder infection, this urine sample will be sterile. If you do have bacteria in your bladder, the urine sample should test positive for bacteria. Moreover, the culture test will indicate which bacteria are causing the infection and how significant the bacterial invasion and growth may be. The bacteria that most commonly cause cystitis are *E. coli,* enterococcus, *E. coli* and strept fecalis. Your physician will prescribe a different medication for the different types of bacteria.

The number of bacteria in both your bladder and in the laboratory doubles every few hours. The severity of an infection can depend on what is called the *inoculum*—how many bacteria get into your bladder initially. If you have vaginitis at the time of intercourse, more bacteria might be introduced into your bladder than otherwise. If your inoculum was 50,000 "bugs," it would increase to 100,000 in a short time. But if the inoculum was 5,000 "bugs," it would increase to 10,000, then 20,000, then 40,000, and so on. The smaller the inoculum, the longer it takes for the infection to increase.

In my practice, I recommend patients take three pills of a cephalosporin (Keflex, Ceclor (Aust.), Ceporex) or sulfonamide/ trimethoprim combination (Bactrim, Septrim) all at once to knock out an infection. Unlike many doctors, I do not prescribe a ten-day course of antibiotics for uncomplicated urinary tract infections because I do not think such a condition warrants long-term treatment. As long as the bladder is capable of normal function and empties properly, you should feel better in a few hours.

My attitude about antibiotics is different from that of many of my colleagues. In fact, when I began my practice I had a problem with some patients referred to me by other doctors. I steadfastly refuse to prescribe antibiotics for long periods except in rare exceptions. I also require that patients return in a few days to give a urine sample for a repeat culture.

Some patients reacted to my treatment as if I were asking for the moon. Some women were insecure with my approach because "no one else did it." I explained my reasoning: The bladder is a reservoir. The antibiotic quickly reaches the site where it is needed. A large single dose works to knock out infection rapidly and effectively. Why expose your entire body as well as sensitive bladder tissue to ten days of antibiotic therapy? To me, that didn't make sense.

Some patients, however, finding they couldn't talk me into giving them the drug for ten days, would call their old physicians to get a two-week supply of an antibiotic. The doctors would comply, thinking I must have made a mistake.

However, several infectious disease studies have shown that a single dose of antibiotics eradicates uncomplicated infections with complete safety. This approach, which makes a lot of sense to me, also eliminates the complications of yeast infections and diarrhea that some women develop when taking antibiotics for ten days.

Recently, one of my patients, Pat, confronted her gynecologist. She told me, "I asked him why he insisted on giving me a ten-day course of medication for each bladder infection. Why couldn't I take one or two days of medicine and then come back for a repeat culture to see if bacteria were still in my bladder? He said he couldn't do that because patients would not want to return to his office and pay fifty dollars for a second culture. I was furious," Pat said. "I told him he was not giving women a choice."

After a while, I managed to persuade most of my patients to adopt this common sense approach to treating bacterial infections of the bladder. They have come to learn that antibiotics are not a safe panacea. Antibiotics are miraculous drugs that have a central role in medicine. But they should not be abused by patient or physician alike.

As all my patients do, Tricia came to my office three days after taking the antibiotic—recovered and rested, but with her recent activities still fresh in her mind—so that we could figure out together what caused her problem. Her first urine culture had grown one organism, confirming that it was a genuine bacterial infection. (If it had been sterile, we would have had to figure out other causes of her symptoms.) When she came back, we took a second urine sample to make sure her urine was normal and free of infection.

Some patients continue to feel the symptoms of burning and frequency several days after the medication is finished, even though the bacteria are gone. This is because the bladder lining needs time to recuperate after bacterial attack. You should not take a second course of antibiotics just because you still feel symptoms. Get a second culture and prove there are living bacteria in your urine before you expose yourself to more drugs. Symptoms of irritation often will be relieved by taking pyridium (a prescription bladder analgesic) or a teaspoon of baking soda in water.

Just one bladder infection is a sign that something is wrong with your "voiding unit." There are certainly many ways this unit can fail. If your food processor has ever broken you know there could be something wrong with the blade, pusher, chopper, switch, wiring, or other components. Similarly, there are numerous things that can go wrong with your urinary tract. Figuring out the reason is an exercise in problem solving. We need to examine all the possibilities and eliminate the ones that don't make sense for your situation.

A Visit to My Office: Six Questions for Tracking Down the Cause of an Infection

When Tricia came into my office, she filled out a questionnaire to help us decipher what caused her infection. I wanted to know everything that she had ever observed about her urologic history. Each of the questions that follows relates to a different aspect of my theories about the causes of cystitis. All my patients are given this questionnaire when they first visit my office, and the answers to these questions provide valuable clues in the search for the cause of bouts with cystitis.

1. *Do you have a history of urinary tract infections as a child?*
2. *When did your first infection develop?*
3. *What methods of birth control have you used and when?*
4. *When did you last have intercourse?*
5. *Do you have frequent vaginal infections?*
6. *Do you have a good stream when you void, particularly after intercourse?*

Question 1: Do You Have a History of Urinary Tract Infections?

If you had infections as a child, it tells me you may have a true anatomic problem. Since anatomic causes are so rare, however, I would want to eliminate other possible factors before putting you through tests that examine your anatomy.

Question 2: When Did Your First Infection Develop?

The timing of your first infection gives me clues about the cause of your present one.

For example, for many women, their first urinary tract infections occurred with the onset of sexual activity. This can be a problem for teenage girls who develop cystitis but who don't want their mothers to know they are sexually active. Girls who don't seek help for their symptoms right away can damage sensitive bladder tissue and cause themselves even more grief. Cystitis, in fact, is often called "honeymoon cystitis" because it often appeared in young women who were just married and sexually active for the first time in their lives. Today, of course, mores have changed and many young women have sexual relations before they have a honeymoon. The woman who develops cystitis upon the first exposure to intercourse may have something wrong with how her bladder functions. Or there may be some problem traceable to how she is performing intercourse.

On the other hand, there are women who have intercourse for years and never develop a bladder infection, then suddenly get one. This situation points to a change in the system and makes functional problems more suspect, for we know their systems worked fine right up to a certain point. Then we investigate what happened to make the change occur.

This question of whether you were able to have intercourse without getting infections or whether the infections began the moment you started having intercourse is important because it helps me determine if the symptoms are related to a functional or an anatomic cause or some combination of both.

Question 3: What Methods of Birth Control Have You Used and When?

I ask this question because I have found that some women who use diaphragms are susceptible to urinary tract infections.

It was a very observant patient who first said to me, "You know, I think it's my diaphragm that's causing me to get these infections." This immediately piqued my interest. Here was one distinct difference between myself (who has never had a urinary tract infection) and this patient: I had never used a diaphragm.

Could this widely used method of birth control be an accomplice in recurrent urinary tract infections? This connection had not been studied, and I decided to find out. I designed a study that would confirm or deny my suspicions.

THE DIAPHRAGM STUDY:
THE DIAPHRAGM-CYSTITIS LINK

The first step was the selection of patients. One hundred fifty women who had recurrent urinary tract infections agreed to participate. They were otherwise healthy and had no history of urinary tract infections in childhood and had never had vaginal or bladder surgery.

I asked them the same questions about their sexual activity and use of birth control. Ninety-four percent said they thought their infections were related to sexual intercourse. And 87 percent said their infections began only after they had become sexually active. A quarter of them had had recurrent vaginal infections with their bladder infections. And two out of three reported they had a poor urine stream after intercourse but a strong forceful one at all other times.

Of the 150 women in the study, 102 used a diaphragm. Each of these 102 came back to the office wearing her diaphragm and had the uroflow and residual urine check redone.

Interestingly, I found that when they wore their diaphragms, their urine flow rates changed dramatically. The pressure of their urine flow was lower and their bladders took longer to empty.

To make this a proper scientific study, I had to find out if one factor—the fitting of the diaphragm—was consistent. If the devices were fitted very differently, it would make other correlations less credible.

So, in the tradition of medical experimentation, I participated in my own study. I learned the names of all the specialists who had fitted the diaphragm wearers in my study. There were fourteen of them, gynecologists and nurse practitioners, all in the Los Angeles area. I called each one and made an appointment to have myself fitted with a diaphragm.

When visiting their offices, I did not tell them the purpose of my study. I knew confidentiality would be maintained and that they would not find out I had visited each one as part of an experiment.

Diaphragm sizes are measured in millimeters. An 80-millimeter diaphragm is large and a 65-millimeter diaphragm is considered small. At the fourteen fittings, I received thirteen 80-millimeter diaphragms and one 75-millimeter diaphragm.

Unfortunately, all fourteen were far too big for my small frame.

Back in the office, I compared my urine flow rate with and without the diaphragms. My normal average flow rate is 18 cubic centimeters of urine per second. With an 80-millimeter diaphragm it dropped to 12 to 13 cubic centimeters per second. This drop suggested that obstruction was occurring.

What does this finding mean? As shown in my patients, the diaphragms as fitted by most health specialists tend to reduce normal flow rates (see illustration). The devices were literally obstructing normal urine flow by putting pressure on the bladder neck. In some patients, the diaphragm restricted urine flow by as much as 40 percent by altering the angle of the bladder neck. This means that urine could easily be left in the bladder along with bacteria from recent sexual intercourse. Since most women keep the diaphragm in place up to eight hours after intercourse, you can see how easy it might be for an infection to arise.

My patients found they had to squeeze very hard to fully empty their bladders when wearing their diaphragms. Without the dia-

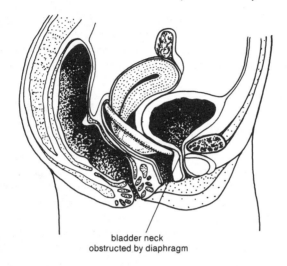

bladder neck
obstructed by diaphragm

Figure 1-3, Bladder Neck Obstructed by a Diaphragm

phragms, their flow rates were perfectly normal; no urine was left in their bladders.

For example, one patient's normal flow left 2 cubic centimeters of residual urine in her bladder after voiding—essentially nothing. With an 80-millimeter flat-spring diaphragm, 40 cubic centimeters (about one-sixth of a cup) was left over and with a 75-millimeter flat-spring diaphragm, 34 cubic centimeters were left in her bladder.

Now, all these diaphragms were "properly fitted" by competent gynecologists and nurse practitioners. But after seeing the bladder neck obstruction produced in so many of my patients, I began to question the notion of what is considered "proper fit."

One popular book on women's health care written by a doctor asserts that using the largest possible correctly fitting size insures that the diaphragm will not be displaced during intercourse. But what is "correctly fitting"?

In essence you should not be able to feel the diaphragm once it is in place. Doctors and nurses are taught to fit diaphragm users with the "largest comfortable size." But for many women, this means that, inside the vagina, the coil-spring rim that gives the diaphragm its shape presses snugly against the pubic bone. When the diaphragm fits that tightly, it presses on the bladder neck. During intercourse, the diaphragm rim rubs and may irritate the bladder neck.

Many physicians will tell you that a diaphragm is a barrier method of birth control. That is, that the device itself blocks the entry of sperm into the cervix. I do not subscribe to this idea. Sperm are minuscule; we need a microscope to see even one. It simply is not possible to bar them completely from entering the cervix with a rubber disc. I tell patients, "They'll pole vault over the thing if they want to." So it does no good to make diaphragms fit tightly. It would take a diaphragm the size of a newborn baby's head to make a completely occlusive barrier.

Rather, I believe the diaphragm should be viewed as a receptacle for spermicide. In fact, Masters and Johnson have shown in their studies of sexuality that during intercourse the vagina expands and contracts. During intercourse, every diaphragm floats around somewhat, even the ones that fit tightly when the vagina is in a resting state. (Since the male penis comes in all sizes and most women can accommodate the differences, it seems logical that a diaphragm of a smaller size would also be snugly held in place by good vaginal tone.)

Since the diaphragm is meant only to hold spermicide in place so that any sperm will be less likely to get by, a properly fitted diaphragm does not have to be as "large as can be accommodated" (see illustration).

It is critically important, however, that you put your diaphragm in correctly. The spermicide goes inside the cup and the cup rests against the cervix. As each thrust of the penis against the diaphragm pushes more spermicide into the cervical opening, the cervix becomes coated with the sperm-killing substance. This is what makes the device so effective.

My diaphragm-wearing patients continued the experiment for another year. I fitted most of them with a smaller diaphragm, the largest one that did not cause obstruction to the bladder neck but still covered the cervix. This usually turned out to be a 65-millimeter one. When inserted, the practitioner should be able to fit a portion of his or her finger between the spring and the vagina.

How can you tell if your diaphragm is the correct size? Very

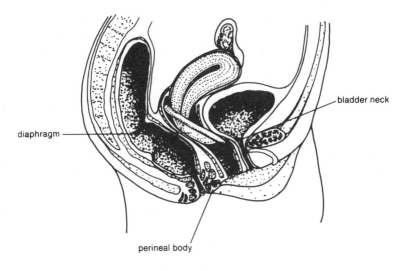

Figure 1-4, A Properly Fitted Diaphragm

simply: You should *never* be able to feel the diaphragm once it is in place. If you do, it is too big. It should not obstruct the bladder neck.

How do you feel for your bladder neck? Put your forefinger inside your vagina. Press up against the pubic bone and roll your finger back and forth. You will feel a tube. That is your urethra. Follow the tube further up your vagina until you feel a V shape. That is your bladder neck.

After one year, all but one whose diaphragms were refitted were free of infection. Six women did not follow my recommendation to change diaphragm size and they still had infections. Others switched birth control methods and were infection-free. Three followed recommendations but continued to experience infections for other reasons.

The startling discovery from this study was that, for diaphragm wearers, simply alleviating obstruction caused by too large a diaphragm or switching the method of birth control stopped recurrent urinary tract infections.

Thus, if you are trying to track down the cause of your infection and you use a diaphragm, the first thing I would advise you to do is to be certain your diaphragm is not obstructing the easy flow of urine. You don't have to give up the diaphragm; just get a smaller size. As my study shows, your risk of pregnancy is not likely to increase, and your risk of repeated cystitis may be eliminated. Studies have shown that the failure of the diaphragm to be an effective contraceptive method is based more on the "diaphragm in the drawer" syndrome than on improper fit.

I don't want to frighten you from using the diaphragm. In fact, just in the last year I switched to this method of birth control myself because I have reached the age when the pill is no longer recommended. I have not had a bladder infection. Rest assured, the diaphragm is an excellent method of birth control. It is safe and effective and has fewer side effects than any other method.

A good way to prevent infections is to void before you insert the diaphragm and have intercourse. Do not void again until you have to, so that you generate a good, efficient stream. If six hours have passed since intercourse, remove the diaphragm and then void. By removing the obstruction, you allow your bladder to function as nature intended.

Many doctors today advise cystitis patients to void right before and right after intercourse to prevent infection. This is not correct. You should not urinate after intercourse until you feel the need. You should wait until you can void with a forceful stream, for a few drops of urine dribbling out after intercourse is no protection at all. Your bladder should be at least half full. You can influence this cleansing mechanism by drinking fluids just before or after intercourse, thus assuring that you will have to urinate within a few hours. Remember, it's not simply the fact that you void after intercourse that counts. You have to void with some force to cleanse your urinary tract of any bacteria that might have been introduced during intercourse.

If you continue having problems with your diaphragm, you might consider alternate methods of birth control. Aside from the pill and IUD, which some women avoid due to side effects, other methods are available. Cervical caps and sponges are gaining popularity but must be used according to directions to avoid vaginal infections. If you have had all the children you want and find birth control methods problematic, consider a tubal ligation for you or a vasectomy for your spouse.

Four Steps for a Healthy Bladder

To keep your bladder healthy, you must empty it efficiently. This "mechanical" function is dependent on four factors:

• The amount of residual urine left in the bladder after voiding.
• The rate of urinary flow—that is, how forceful your stream is.
• The frequency of voiding; the less often you void, the longer urine stays in your bladder.
• The rate of bacterial multiplication, which depends on how large the initial introduction of bacteria into the bladder was.

These factors are implicated in cystitis. For example, the diaphragm can affect each one. It can increase residual urine by obstructing the bladder neck and decrease the rate of urinary flow. If you jump up after intercourse to void, your bladder may not be half full and capable of generating a good, forceful stream. Your stream should be capable of moving dirt on a sidewalk. If it can't move dirt, it's not forceful enough. Finally, if the diaphragm stays in for a long time, bacteria can stay in the bladder long enough to multiply into hazardous numbers.

It is still news to many people that the diaphragm has been implicated in urinary tract infections. When I first began my study, I didn't think it was so unusual. One day I was driving a friend, who is a professor of pediatric surgery, along with his family and my daughter, to Disneyland. When I mentioned the link between cystitis and diaphragms he turned to me, surprised, and said, "My God, that's an interesting concept. Maybe that's what I'm seeing in my teenage patients." That was the first time I began to think that what I was doing was different.

At that point, I entered my scientific study in an essay competition sponsored by the Western region of the American Urological Association. I won honorable mention in the contest, beaten out only by a study on penile implants and another on prostate cancer.

My scientific article on the diaphragm was not published until a full two years after I had assembled the data and made the conclusions. In the world of research, this is a normal delay. It takes time to design a study, carry it out, write it, submit it, and then wait for other experts to referee it. If those experts find fault with a study, the author must convincingly counter those criticisms before the study is published. My study sailed through this process, but it still took two years.

After I put together the scientific study, I wrote a popular article for a well-known woman's magazine. But the magazine refused to run it without making major changes—recommended by other doctors—that would have completely changed my conclusions. The magazine editors believed the article was too controversial because, in the minds of the doctors they consulted, the link was not yet "proven" and "wasn't true."

I demanded the article back and then submitted it to *Ms.* magazine, which published it without changing a word. The editors stood behind every point. *Ms.*, which considers itself on the cutting edge of women's problems, had the courage to take something that made sense and put it forth as a major health finding.

After the *Ms.* article appeared, I was called by editors of other magazines and by television producers who were excited about the new findings. By appearing on television, I found that I could get my message to a wide audience in a short time.

The response was very positive. At television studios, while sitting in the so-called green room before going on the air, women always approached me to discuss in private their urinary tract problems. They poured out their stories, and were starved for information about cystitis, incontinence, and other urologic problems.

As I listened, I realized women were not getting information about urology. They had painful bladder infections and didn't know what to do about them. They leaked urine when they sneezed and didn't know why. But no one was talking about such problems.

On one show, there was a great debate before airtime over whether or not I should use the word *vagina*. Evidently, no one had ever used this word on the program. The staff had agreed that "vagina" would not be mentioned on the air. But I simply refused to talk to the audience as if they were children. There is no reason not to use correct terminology in discussing female health problems.

When I did use the word "vagina," I saw smiles cross the faces of the cameraperson and sound technician, both of whom were women, as this forbidden word was finally spoken.

On another show, I discussed diaphragms. This word was also taboo, but I ignored the rules and even showed an illustration of a diaphragm. The reaction of the studio audience was not one of shock, dismay, or disgust. Rather, after my segment on the show, they kept asking for more information. They commended the television producers for discussing—at last—issues that needed to be aired. Vaginas and diaphragms, the television producers realized, are not dark secrets. They are normal parts of life. These shows led to other appearances during which I talked about incontinence. It seems once we got past diaphragms, we could go on to that taboo.

Meanwhile, my study has been replicated and corroborated by other researchers. Doctors at the University of Washington recently found that women who use diaphragms have a rate of bladder infections four times greater than that of women who use other methods of birth control. Both the scientific article and the *Ms.* article on the diaphragm-cystitis link are often cited by other researchers because of their early significance.

What might be done to make diaphragms more compatible with a woman's body? Aside from using smaller diaphragms, the

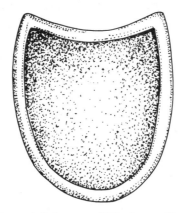

Figure 1-5, Improved Diaphragm Design

device might be designed differently. I have suggested one possibility, a diaphragm that uses a soft wire at the point where the device encounters the bladder neck (see Figure 1-5). It is a simple change, and such a diaphragm would not put undue pressure on the bladder neck and it would always fit in just one way. A wearer would always know it was properly and securely in place. Unfortunately, the companies that make diaphragms still consult gynecologists who think the diaphragm should be a "snug" barrier method. It seems we still have a long way to go in convincing others to improve women's urologic health.

Question 4: When Did You Last Have Intercourse?

Of course, not all women who use diaphragms get bladder infections and not everyone who gets cystitis uses a diaphragm. What about my other patients?

Clues can be taken from answers to the fourth question on my questionnaire, for certain aspects of intercourse can lead to a urinary tract infection.

A little-regarded fact is the impact of sexual positions on urethral trauma and bladder infections. Many men, it seems, receive their sexual education from magazines like *Penthouse* and *Playboy*. Their photographs often depict men in a very dominant position for intercourse. The man is raised at arm's length above the woman, apparently ready to conquer all.

Unfortunately for women, men are not built to make this a satisfactory position. The penis is normally suspended at a 45-degree angle from the man's abdominal wall. When he enters from on high, in what we might call the dominating missionary position, his anatomy forces him to thrust with a corkscrew up and down motion. This motion drags the urethra up and down in the vagina and the urethra quickly becomes sore and swollen. Abrasions can make bacteria adhere more easily.

This dominant position is extremely unhealthy and unsatisfying (see illustration). The vagina has a "G spot," or erogenous zone, along its top wall. The other erogenous spot, the clitoris, is outside the vagina. If the male enters at a lower angle, the natural alignment is such that the clitoris is compressed and the G spot is massaged. He performs a rocking motion which is more stimulating for both partners and the female urethra is spared unnecessary stress.

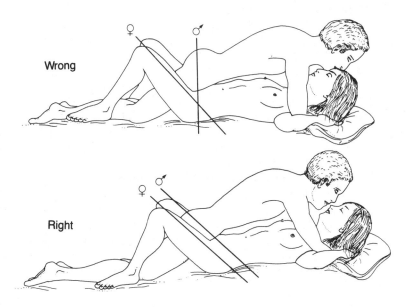

Figure 1-6, Right and Wrong Positions for Intercourse

No sexual position is inherently dangerous. Rather it is alignment—the angle of the penis against the vagina—that counts. No position will damage the urethra if this alignment is correct.

Using spermicides for intercourse may be to blame for your infection. While they may be helpful in killing harmful bacteria (such as gonorrhea) in the vagina, excess amounts of chemicals can harm vaginal or urethral tissues. This is especially true of the foaming spermicides that are inserted as tablets into the vaginal opening. The foam can chemically burn the vagina or urethra, making it red, swollen, and tender to the touch. Other spermicides come in a cream base that is kinder than foams. When inserted with applicators, the spermicide is right up on the cervix where it is expected to work.

In any case, don't use too much spermicide. Excess cream or foam will spread outside the vagina and become a potential carrier for bacteria. This is also true of lubricants such as K-Y Lubricating Jelly or Vaseline petroleum jelly that some couples use to moisten the penis before intercourse. If you use gobs of lubricant, you are providing gobs of a viscous material on which bacteria can hitch a ride and grow.

A safer way to use K-Y Jelly is to put it on sparingly, where you need it. Put some on the tip of your index finger and open your labia with your other hand. Place the jelly on the back portion of the vagina's opening (see illustration). This is the point where the penis creates friction and drag. If you are not lubricated by your own natural secretions or if your tissue is dry because of lack of estrogen, you can experience lacerations and tears to the vagina at this point, called the *posterior forchette*. By lubricating this place with a dab of jelly, you will prevent harmful friction and will minimize the amount of jelly that can spread beyond your vaginal canal and into the urethra.

Infrequent sex is *not* a factor in cystitis, as some doctors may have you believe. Rather, the problem lies in the lack of lubrication. If you are relaxed and your naturally lubricating vaginal fluids are secreted during foreplay, intercourse should not cause friction and damage your vagina or urethra.

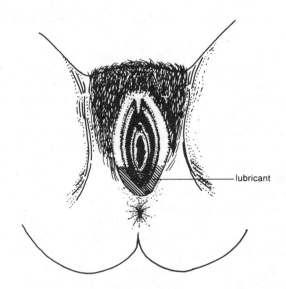

Figure 1-7, Proper Lubricant Placement for Women

Contrary to popular belief, oral sex is not a cause of cystitis either. Your partner's "germs" have nothing to do with your cystitis. In my six years of practice, I've never found a "strange" throat organism in the urine being tested for bacteria. There is simply no basis for the old wives' tale that oral sex causes bladder infections.

Nor is there any basis for the belief that venereal disease is a precursor to cystitis. The two are not related. This old wives' tale may stem from a subtle male orientation that promiscuous women must get bladder infections. Not so.

Sexually transmitted bacterial infections such as trichomonas and chlamydia can cause symptoms of irritation leading to vaginitis and urethritis, however. Chlamydia is now thought to be present in the cervix of about 10 percent of sexually active women in America, especially those under twenty-two who have had herpes or other genital infections. Often, a woman infected with chlamydia has no symptoms. Her gynecologist may notice a mucous discharge on her cervix and that is all. When cultured, the mucus is shown to carry a cervical chlamydia infection.

Trichomonas is easily detected by looking at a smear of vaginal fluid under a microscope. The organism has a characteristic size and shape, including little tails, or flagelli. Gonorrhea and syphilis are long-recognized venereal diseases which require treatment for both partners.

If you have these symptoms and your urine culture is negative for showing bacteria in your bladder, you should probably be screened for these sexually transmitted bacteria because they are increasingly common. One woman was told by her physician that she had a "scaly urethra" when no bacteria were found in her urine culture. In actuality, she had urethritis induced by chlamydia.

Unlike nonspecific urethritis and urinary tract infection, which cannot be sexually transmitted, trichomonas, chlamydia, gonorrhea, and syphilis require that both partners take an antibiotic.

But now, what if you have a normal flow rate, don't use a diaphragm, and still get infections? We will continue to look for reasons with help from the fifth question.

Question 5: Do you have frequent vaginal infections?

Vaginitis arises when the protective layer of tissue found on the vagina and urethra becomes decreased or absent for any reason. Normally, the layer protects sensitive tissue from bacteria. But when it is rubbed away, bacteria can invade the urethra. There is itching, discharge, burning inside the vagina, and burning on the outside of the urethra when you urinate. There may also be a mild feeling of frequency and urgency.

Since vaginitis is essentially increased bacterial growth in the vagina, it can lead to cystitis.

Using a diaphragm can lead to a vaginal infection. Since it is a foreign body, it can irritate the vagina. If left in the vagina longer than the recommended six to eight hours, the risk of vaginitis increases. If you forget and leave your diaphragm in for a day, I recommend that you douche with a mild vinegar and water solution (one tablespoon to one quart water) to restore the normal acid-alkaline balance in the vagina.

A seemingly ridiculous but common cause of vaginitis and urethritis is designer jeans or pants that are too tight for the build of your body. The center seam rubs your perineal skin and abrades the tissue so that bacteria can adhere. Irritation follows. I do not have one of those elite designer-jean bodies, but I would caution you about trying to maintain that image. If the center seam pulls up on your labia when you sit and you have that tight, drawn-up feeling between the labia, the urethra, and the rectum, those are not the kinds of jeans you should be wearing.

Women who are prone to vaginal yeast infections often get the symptoms of cystitis. Such women tend to have abnormal sugar metabolism—either too much, as in diabetes, or too little, as in hypoglycemia. If you binge on sugar, you may set yourself up for yeast infections, and yeast in the urethra is very irritating. When this happens, you may feel that you have a bladder infection when in fact you don't. This is another example of why urine cultures are so important. If you frequently take antibiotics in the absence of infection, you are setting yourself up for potentially chronic bladder problems. In fact, antibiotics may actually damage your bladder and exacerbate the symptoms of cystitis. Many antibiotics cause upset stomachs, alter normal bowel metabolism, and make you even more susceptible to vaginal yeast infections.

Another source of infection in the vagina and the urethra is an allergy to the materials used in commercially available tampons and pads. Women with this allergy tend to get symptoms in the third day after their menstrual period begins. These women may make their own pads out of cloth rather than fiber, but then the problem is that cotton cloth does not carry blood away from the inner part of the pad, which is the part near the vagina. Bacteria grow in blood and are kept next to the urethra, and this easily irritates the urethra and causes urethritis, or inflammation of the urethra. I know one woman who solves this dilemma by making her own cotton pads by wrapping them in Handiwipes. Handiwipes are similar to the wrappings on menstrual pads that carry blood from the outside to the cotton inside. If you have to make your own pads for any reason, such as an allergy or because you are too large to wear commercially made pads, use Handiwipes to help protect you from infection.

I once had a patient come to me because she was developing a culture-proven bladder infection every month. This woman, who was a high-powered executive, did not wear a diaphragm and had had intercourse for many years without ever getting infections. Her infections were in no way related to intercourse. We could not figure out what caused them until one day she said, "You know, the infection always happens by the third to fourth day of my period." I instantly realized how she could solve her problem. She was getting infections because she had switched to super-absorbent tampons, which tended, as they expanded, to obstruct her bladder neck. She would void two or three times before removing the high-capacity tampon. As soon as she started pulling the tampon out every time she urinated, she was infection-free and no longer had cystitis.

Once a nurse told me that her sister had chronic bladder infections that arose on the third day of her period each month. The infections had invaded the sister's kidneys on several occasions so that doctors had prescribed chronic antibiotic suppressive therapy. I told the nurse to tell her sister to pull out her tampons every time she voided. The infections stopped.

Again, this was a common sense "cure" to cystitis that you could figure out by yourself. You've got to observe your habits and environment. Focus on everything you can. You are a partner in mystery solving every time you visit a physician.

If you wear tampons, I recommend that you make it a habit to pull one out each time you void. They are not expensive and the practice will keep your bladder neck and urethra free from obstruction. Next time you wear a tampon, listen to your flow and hear how it slows your urine stream as you void.

Question 6: Do You Have a Good Stream When You Void?

If your recent bladder infection did not come about after sexual activity or as a result of a vaginal infection, we have to look for other causes. The answer to the last question on my questionnaire can shed light on the matter: Do you have a good stream when you void?

Put another way, when you are in a public ladies' room, does your urinary flow rate sound as good as that of the woman in the next stall? Do you empty your bladder as quickly as your girlfriend does?

By paying attention, you may save yourself considerable trouble in the future. When Sarah came to see me last year, she was doubly perturbed. In recent years, she was having to urinate more and more frequently. "It built up gradually," she explained. "Eventually I couldn't wait an hour before having to go again. I found myself preoccupied with bathrooms. I chose dark clothing so that if I had an accident, no one would notice. Finally I got fed up and decided to get help."

Sarah went to her gynecologist, a woman physician, and explained her problem. The physician, recalling her training, said Sarah needed an operation to tighten the ligaments under her bladder and to remove her uterus. The reasoning: The ligaments had been stretched, and even if they were tightened, the uterus would make them fall again. This, the doctor said, was why Sarah had to urinate frequently.

Sarah said she was appalled at this news. "I don't know the long-term consequences of a hysterectomy. Major surgery is risky. I was in a real dilemma. I felt my doctor was wiser than me. But the urinary problem was unbearable. My girlfriend was a patient of Dr. Gillespie's, so I called for an appointment to see if something else could be done."

When Sarah came to see me for a second opinion, we tested her flow rate. Sure enough, it was sluggish. Her stream was not forceful and her bladder never emptied itself fully. She kept having to urinate sooner and more often. Many women with this problem develop recurrent urinary tract infections. But Sarah was luckier. Her major symptom was frequency.

The cause could be traced to the nerves in her lower back. Without realizing it, Sarah had damaged a disc, which compressed the nerves that signal her bladder to void. Her nerves were "shorted out."

"I was really surprised," Sarah said. "I felt only minimal back pain. Otherwise I was fine. I didn't exercise and I do wear high heels. Something had thrown my back out."

Sarah took a medication that stimulated these nerves to fire properly. "Within forty-eight hours," she said, "I felt relief. Gradually, I have been taking less and less medicine because I've been taking care of my back with proper exercises. I watch how I sit and lift and I threw away my spike heels. I'm almost off medication now and my flow rate is normal. The thing that astonishes me is that I almost let someone take out my uterus, when all I needed was physical therapy and a few pills temporarily."

I often hear from patients that their streams are intermittent and tend to flow in spurts instead of in a smooth pattern. There is considerable straining to get all the urine out.

If this sounds like you, a uroflow exam could identify that you have a primary bladder problem. It will tell us if your bladder is

---

A Uroflow Exam

A uroflow is simply a graph of how you void. As you urinate, it charts out—on paper—a graph of your flow rate. Actually, your perception of what is normal may be limited. A uroflow pictures your voiding pattern and eliminates misconceptions. It allows me to compare my flow rate, which is normal, with yours. If your flow rate is abnormal, the uroflow chart will show you the difference.

If you have an abnormal uroflow, it is likely that you will get bladder infections whether or not you have intercourse.

unable to empty efficiently. Remember, it takes a good flow to cleanse bacteria from the bladder and to wash off the perineum and vagina. Residual urine is susceptible to bacterial invasion from your own body even if you are celibate.

BACK PAIN AND UROLOGIC PROBLEMS

There are numerous reasons why your bladder might not empty efficiently. One of the most common is lower back stress in women. You may be going to a gymnasium or exercising at home without proper supervision. If you lift weights you may injure your lower back without knowing it. You may use a rowing machine that puts stress on the lower back muscles.

You may wear heels that are too high for your hip and leg structure. This will cause you to sway your back and increase pressure on your lower spine. The medical term for this swaying of the back to compensate for high heels, pregnancy, or other imbalancers is *lordosis*. It is just one reason why many women suffer bladder dysfunction.

A recent study indicated that from 70 to 90 percent of the United States population will have low back pain at some point in their lives. Lower back pain is the number one cause of disability in people under forty-five and the number three cause in those over forty-five, according to orthopedic surgeons.

Lower back pain is also a leading cause of urinary tract infections in women. This fact is rarely addressed at urology meetings and few physicians have taken the trouble of studying the relationship in detail. Nevertheless, the fact that lower back damage can cause bladder infections has long been known by urologists everywhere.

Why is it so often overlooked? I can only guess that subtle biases may be at work. Gone are the days when lower back pain in a woman was automatically attributed to a "tipped uterus" (such a condition is extremely rare), but many doctors fail to look for other causes of lower back pain in women. Some seem to believe that women have a lower incidence of lower back injury because women tend to lift fewer heavy objects than men. But this is not the case. Women strain their backs just as often as men.

Some physicians are trained to look for overt injury to major nerves in the lower back before making a diagnosis of back injury. But there are many fine nerves in this network that can become strained and then contribute to bladder problems. Indeed, orthopedists in studying patients have found that a certain percentage of people who complain of minor backaches tend to go on to develop ruptured discs. It appears that vague back pains can be indicative of changes in disc support, presaging more serious trouble.

The point is that the bladder can pick up signs of back trouble long before there is more obvious damage to the nerves and discs.

When Irene came to see me, she had been having repeated bladder infections for three years. They came upon her at any time with or without intercourse. Irene constantly took antibiotics. Whenever she stopped, she got another infection. A culture was not taken every time, but when it was, it showed that her problem was with genuine bacterial infections.

I asked her to give me a uroflow, the first she had ever had done. It showed a severe abdominal straining pattern. Her bladder muscle was not working properly. Upon probing, I found she had an achy lower back. To Irene, it was a minor discomfort, but I convinced her to have X-rays taken of her spine. They showed a major instability of the fifth lumbar vertebra. It was the kind of problem that usually requires surgery.

Then it hit her. Her bladder infections began at the same time, three years ago, that she had had a sledding accident. She came down the hill, fell, and landed hard on her tailbone. Her lower back was injured, creating her bladder problem. If someone had given her a uroflow when her infections first began, she could have avoided years of taking antibiotics and having recurrent infections.

Indeed, the bladder is the most sensitive indicator of lower back problems. Helen, a forty-five-year-old accountant, had bladder problems for three weeks. Her uroflow showed abdominal straining. I told her that I suspected it was her back. She laughed, saying her back felt fine. Then, one day, she called to say she was in traction. She had a slowly moving disc which did not hurt until it had slipped a certain amount. But it had caused bladder problems immediately and was a sure sign of impending back trouble.

Nina is an artist who does silk-screening at a nearby university. As she leaned over her table, reaching for supplies, she strained her back and began developing bladder infections. Once she learned to stand straight, her bladder got better. Studies have shown that when you sit, the pressure on your lower discs is 40 percent greater than when you stand. Thus people who have sedentary jobs—artists, secretaries, writers—have a higher incidence of disc rupture than do people who stand and walk around on their jobs.

Virginia, an avid gardener, gets cystitis every spring. "It's because I sit on the cold ground," she believed. "It weakens my bladder." But Virginia also has a lower back problem. Every spring, when she goes out to start her garden, she strains her back and initiates cystitis. It has nothing to do with sitting on cold ground.

A large group of nerves to the bladder originate in your lower spine between two vertebrae (see illustration). The point is called the *lumbar fourth and fifth interspace*. Compression in this area shorts out the transmission of one of your body's chemical messengers that helps your bladder function. You can think of the bladder as being like a battery. The nerves leading to the battery from your lower back are like battery cables. And the chemical, called *acetylcholine,* is like the battery acid. If the cable cannot transmit enough current, the charge in the battery does not build up enough to start the car—in this case to generate a normal, efficient bladder contraction.

Injury or damage to the nerves of your lower back may impair the transmission of "current" to your bladder. Like a weak battery, the bladder does not function well. It does not empty efficiently and may leave residual urine, which can lead to infections. This type of infection is best treated with a longer course of antibiotics. Depending on the individual, the drug may be needed for five to seven days.

The condition can be corrected in two ways. One is to give you bethanechol chloride (a synthetic acetylcholine) on a daily basis. The extra chemical, commonly used in your body as a neurotransmitter to help nerves "fire," aids in restoring normal bladder function. A second approach is to resolve your lower back stress. Many of my patients stop having bladder infections once they discover how they are straining their backs.

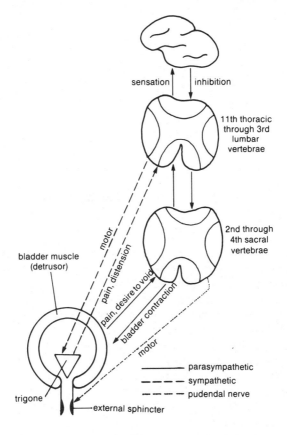

Figure 1-8, Nerve Network to the Bladder

Compare in the diagram on page 46 my uroflow with the uroflow of a patient with lower back injury. Mine is a smooth bell-shaped curve, like a smoothly accelerating and decelerating automobile. Hers is a zigzag shape, like a car that is lugging with loss of power.

If this appears to be your problem we can help resolve it by giving you a single X-ray. If we see a narrowing between the discs where these nerves to the bladder originate, or any evidence of instability, we know you have a physical problem that will benefit

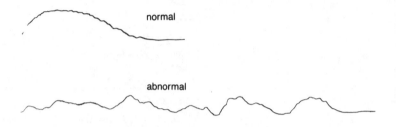

Figure 1-9, Normal and Abnormal Uroflows

by intense physical therapy or orthopedic manipulation. Oral doses of bethanechol chloride can help support neural transmission until the primary problem is resolved.

If you show no damage, we can treat your "silent disc" with stretching exercises such as yoga exercises. Swimming is another excellent exercise that strengthens the back and stomach muscles. If you have access to a gymnasium, lie facedown across the piece of equipment called the horse. Support your stomach and hips and let your legs and toes touch the floor. Then bring your legs up so that your body is horizontal, over the horse. Pull your legs apart and then together before dropping them to the floor. If you do this ten times, you will work the muscles of your lower back in proper alignment. You can also lie on the floor on your back. Bring both knees up to your chest and hold them, while rolling gently from left to right.

If these exercises work, you may not need continuous medication. You can watch your progress when new uroflows are taken. It is truly rewarding to watch the smile on a patient's face when she looks at a successful comparison of her first uroflow and, after some hard work on her part, a later uroflow. The payoff is there, graphically displayed.

Yet another factor in lower back injury is being overweight. If you are carrying ten pounds of extra weight on your stomach, the weight is centered about ten inches in front of your spine. Your back muscles are located two inches behind your spine. To balance this weight, your back muscles must exert a force of fifty pounds to counterbalance the ten pounds on your belly. You can see that just a few pounds extra weight exerts a strain on your back.

Unfortunately, many urologists do not bother to evaluate lower back strain by asking their cystitis patients to take a uroflow exam. Rather, they assume the infection must be sexually related. The lower back simply is not considered. They assume that minor back problems are irrelevant and that only major problems, requiring surgery, could be related to urologic health. As a result, many women are prescribed unnecessary chronic suppressive antibiotic therapy to prevent recurrent urinary tract infections.

HAVE A UROFLOW DONE

A uroflow is useful for making sense of another common misdiagnosis of cystitis patients, that of "the narrow urethra." Almost weekly I see new patients, like Jenny, who tell the same sad story: "My doctor told me I have the urethra of a child," Jenny said. "It was too narrow and too tight so that my urine didn't flow as it should. I needed dilations every six weeks to stretch out and help mature my urethra."

Although the dilations were terribly painful, Jenny said she found she voided better for a few days afterward. "I didn't dare not go back," she said. "He said I would keep getting infections if I didn't come in regularly. I took antibiotics for several days after every dilation. Finally he said I could avoid the inconvenience of regular dilation simply by having surgery which would make it wider."

Is there such a thing as a narrow urethra? The answer is, emphatically, *no*. Incredibly often the poor urethra is blamed for the problem caused by a lazy bladder muscle, which can be traced to lower back problems.

Does it make sense to have your urethra snipped? The answer, again, is no.

When Jenny gave a uroflow, her problem was immediately apparent. She showed a marked inability to achieve a normal flow rate. Her infections could be traced to a bladder that did not contract, not one that could not drain.

Upon examination, her urethra was perfectly normal. For a discussion of why urethral dilations came into vogue and why they have no place in modern urology, please see Chapter Five, "Anatomy Is *Not* Destiny."

Jenny asked why she seemed to void better for a few days after the dilations. The reason is simple: The procedure would paralyze her urethra, which contains muscles to hold in urine. When the muscles are knocked out of action, gravity would drain her lazy bladder and she felt better. The proper treatment for Jenny was exercise to correct her lower back problem and medication to stimulate the muscle to contract fully. She never had another dilation.

A woman recently came to me with bladder infections caused by a highly unusual set of circumstances, and the diagnosis was aided by an examination of her uroflow, which was very odd. The uroflow showed a high ascent curve with straining and then it got sporadic. It appeared that she could generate pressure well enough in the beginning by pushing with her abdominal muscles, but then there were stops and starts that did not seem to reflect that she was straining to urinate. I suspected that she was not relaxing her pelvic floor when she voided.

When I pointed this out to her, she said that her doctor told her that voiding and defecating at the same time was proof that she had a neurologically damaged bladder. He made her practice controlling her anal sphincter by squeezing it when she voided so as to gain control. This would be like doing Kegel vaginal exercises when you need to have a bowel movement. This, of course, is nonsense. But the woman tried so hard to hold back her stool if she was voiding that she never fully emptied her bladder.

We solved her problem with reeducation. She temporarily took medication to increase her bladder contractions and also enrolled in a yoga class to strengthen her lower back. She also practiced a self-regulatory mechanism. As she sat on the toilet, she completely relaxed her buttocks until she felt her vagina drop down. She felt herself relaxing more and more as she subconsciously pictured urine flowing out. After several weeks of practice, her bladder tone improved and she broke her spastic habit. Her cystitis was cured.

This relaxation exercise can be very helpful to women who have experienced chronic urinary tract infections. With an infection, it is extremely painful to urinate. Thus, you hold back, trying to stall off the inevitable pain. Once your infections are arrested, however, you might continue this "learned" response and hold back when you start to void, thus disrupting your normal pattern. Relaxation exercises, practiced at home, can help overcome this fear and restore normal function.

Mysterious Conditions That Can Cause Infection

Finally, what if you don't fit any of these categories? Do you get infections whether or not you have intercourse? Is your back fine, your uroflow normal, your birth control method nonobstructing?

You may have an acquired anatomic reason for your infections. That is, an explanation lies in some change your body has undergone since childhood. For example, there are glands in the urethra, called *Skene's glands,* which produce wetting agents. They help protect your urethra from urine. Skene's glands, however, can become clogged and infected with bacteria. During intercourse the bacteria are "milked out" of the glands. A urine culture may raise the clinical suspicion that this is your problem if you grow bacteria but have no cystitis symptoms, and a test called the *Tratner urethrogram* can confirm the diagnosis. The glands can be excised to stop the condition.

Similarly, a different gland further up on the urethra can become enlarged, causing what is called a *urethral diverticulum.* These glands can become traumatized during childbirth, enlarging and filling with pus. They hold bacteria that constantly seep into the urine. Women with this problem may be prescribed long-term antibiotic therapy. Every time they stop medication, however, the same bacterial organisms reappear in the urine. This condition can be diagnosed with the same test, the Tratner urethrogram, and surgically removed as well.

Another rare acquired condition is chronic pyelonephritis. The kidney may serve as a breeding ground for bacteria because of its spongelike nature. It may be difficult to knock out such infections and, in this instance, longer term antibiotic therapy is called for. To test if bacteria are stemming from the kidney and not the bladder, a catheter is put up each ureter to draw urine directly from the kidneys. If the bladder urine is positive on culture but the kidney ones are not, the problem is a lower tract infection.

Consider the case of Marion, whose infection turned out to be quite dangerous.

Infections Can Be Dangerous

At thirty-two, Marion decided it was time to interrupt her career and have a baby. She consulted her gynecologist, who told her it was a good idea to get off the pill and use a diaphragm for a few months before actually getting pregnant. This would give Marion's body time to adapt to its normal hormonal balance before embarking on pregnancy.

However, the first time Marion used her new diaphragm, she got a bladder infection. A second infection soon followed and, suspecting it to be the culprit, Marion put the diaphragm in the drawer. At that point, she and her husband decided to buy a house. She resumed taking birth control pills for another year and then saw a new gynecologist for advice on when to get pregnant.

The second doctor, who was a woman, gave Marion the same advice about waiting a few months before getting pregnant. She said to Marion, "Doctors have the habit of fitting diaphragms too small. Here's a different size for you that should work fine."

"The new one felt uncomfortable the moment I put it in," Marion said recently. "But I was determined to use it."

During intercourse with the new diaphragm, Marion felt pain in her side. But she simply ignored it.

The following week, she said, "I felt run down and irritable. By Saturday I was achy all over and grumpy. We made love again but used a condom. I just couldn't put the diaphragm in again."

On Saturday afternoon, Marion and her husband went shopping for a new piano. "When we got back, I should have felt elated," she said, "but I felt awful. I began to feel like I was getting a bladder infection. I thought, 'Oh, no! Not on a Saturday.' I went to the bathroom and sure enough there was blood and pain. I knew I had an infection, my third one."

Marion said her husband was sympathetic and suggested they cancel plans to join friends that evening to see a film. "I blew up and screamed at him," she said. "I told him, 'You don't understand women! I'm not sick! It's just a bladder infection!' I was really acting irrationally."

Marion telephoned her doctor and explained the symptoms. "She was extremely reluctant to prescribe an antibiotic over the phone," Marion recalled. "She made me go through my symptoms carefully—the achiness, blood, and pain. Finally, she said it sounded like a true infection and phoned in a prescription. I got the pills and took one at 3:00. But I still didn't feel any better."

At 5:00 Marion and her husband met their friends at the theater. "I sat on the aisle because I had to keep getting up to go to the bathroom," Marion said. "I felt worse and worse. Finally, in the bathroom I began to vomit. My head was hot. I thought I was allergic to the medicine. I was so weak I could hardly stand up.

"By the time we got home, I went to bed and heaped covers over me. I kept shaking. My fever was 102 and I thought it must be the flu. My body hurt so bad I couldn't sleep.

"At seven the next morning," Marion continued, "I knew I needed help. I called the doctor and woke her up. She said, 'It might be a kidney infection. To play it safe, meet me at the hospital in one hour.' I could hardly walk. Everything hurt."

At the hospital on Sunday morning, Marion was given immediate treatment for pyelonephritis. The bacteria in her bladder had worked their way into her kidneys—quietly. She received medication intravenously for a full-blown kidney infection. This is not usually life-threatening, but it can require hospitalization.

Marion said she felt better by the following Friday morning. Yet in the following days and months, her urine still tested as positive for having bacteria. This is because the kidney is very much like a sponge. Tiny abscesses throughout the organ can harbor bacteria long after an acute infection is brought under control. Thus bacteria from Marion's kidneys continued to work their way out of her body for months after her infection.

Another diagnosis you could possibly hear, but one you should beware of, is that your urinary tract infections are caused by polyps of the bladder neck. The polyps are said to act like baffles in that they impede the flow of urine. The polyps are said to create turbulence in the area of the bladder neck and to prevent bacteria from getting out of the bladder. Furthermore, many women are told that these polyps must be cauterized to restore normal bladder function.

Women come to my office after having had these "polyps" surgically removed, with still persisting bladder infections. The reason is simple. The polyps are not the cause of bladder infections but rather the result. When you have a nose cold, your nose secretes mucus. When there is inflammation of the bladder (which may or may not be caused by a bacterial infection), these polyps—more accurately called *pseudopolyps*—may form.

Having these polyps removed makes as much sense as having your nose cauterized every time you have a cold. In other words, the so-called polyps are a reaction to an inflammation, not the cause. They are temporarily caused by swelling of the mucous glands and soon go away naturally.

What if you continue to have symptoms in the absence of bacterial infection; that is, you are told there are no bacteria in your urine. Is there nothing wrong with you? Or could you have another disease? Perhaps you've been told you have urethritis, trigonitis, or an "angry bladder." There is inflammation, you are told, but no infection.

If this sounds like your problem, you may have interstitial cystitis, the topic of the next chapter.

Self-Help Do's and Don'ts for Fighting Cystitis

There are many things you can do for yourself to figure out why you have cystitis. Your doctor can help you but you need to think about your lifestyle and how it might contribute to your infections.

• Whenever you develop symptoms of cystitis—burning, frequency, pressure—get a urine culture as soon as possible. It is extremely important to differentiate between true bacterial infections and symptoms produced by other problems. Leave a urine sample for culturing before starting an antibiotic.

• Vitamin C will increase the burn you feel with cystitis. Cranberry juice is not acidic enough to kill bacteria in urine. The extra calories are not worth it. It is a good idea, however, to drink plenty of water when you have cystitis to help cleanse your system.

• Drink one teaspoon (no more) of baking soda in a glass of water to help ease symptoms.

• Look at different methods of birth control. Consider changing diaphragm sizes if you wear one and can feel it when it's in place.

• You can buy urine sticks from a pharmacist to test your urine for bacteria at home. The sticks are color coded and will show you several measures of urine contents.

• Know how to put your diaphragm in properly to prevent additional bacteria from growing on your urethra. The amount of sexual activity is not the culprit in your infections. You could hang from a chandelier and not get an infection. If you use a diaphragm properly, it does not matter how many times you have intercourse.

• Think about voiding properly and completely after intercourse. The bladder needs to be half full to generate a good contraction. You can drink fluids before or after intercourse. A good stream of urine will cleanse away any bacteria that may have reached your bladder.

• Do not squeeze out a few drops after intercourse and consider that you have reduced your chances of getting a bladder infection.

• Remove any obstructing foreign body before voiding.

• Be kind to your urethra. Avoid sexual positions that compromise your urethra.

• Think very seriously about avoiding repeated urethral dilations, particularly if your lower back and bladder functions have not been evaluated.

• And don't let anyone give you a ten-day course of antibiotics if you have an uncomplicated infection. In general, if your infection can be traced to intercourse, you probably have an uncomplicated infection and can take fewer antibiotics. But if you suffer nerve damage and your bladder is functioning poorly, you may need a longer course of drugs.

• Never take an antibiotic without leaving urine for a culture before you start the drug. Do it at home, do it at a clinic, just do it. You must determine if bacteria are present or not.

• Learn how to give a urine sample. A urinalysis is not enough, by itself, to reveal a bladder infection in women. You can contaminate your urine sample by improper collection.

• If you have back problems, consider avoiding the use of a diaphragm. Start all exercise regimens under proper supervision to strengthen your muscles and help prevent bladder problems.

If you follow these simple guidelines, you should not get cystitis. Use your common sense in figuring out what functional or mechanical thing you are doing that encourages bacteria to stay in your bladder.

TWO

Interstitial Cystitis: The Real Story

On the television saga "Dynasty," the character Fallon Carrington Colby endured dramatic pain and suffering dreamed up weekly by imaginative script writers. Little could those writers imagine, however, the real life pain and suffering experienced daily by the actress who played Fallon, Pamela Sue Martin.

Pamela suffered from interstitial cystitis throughout the years she played Fallon on "Dynasty." There were hours on the set when her bladder burned with "electric shocks." As Pamela now recalls, "I was continually plagued by it the last year on the show. Like any health problem, it was exacerbated by pressure. I ignored it as much as I could. But I was in terrible pain."

Today Pamela is no longer controlled by this crippling disease. Her own story, unlike Fallon's, has had a happy ending. She underwent treatments with me in 1984, and has since been free of interstitial cystitis symptoms. "Once the disease was explained to me," she said, "I understood why everything done to me previously didn't work. I knew what my body had been through and I could now understand why other treatments were ineffectual. Dr. Gillespie's therapy worked. I've been fine ever since and I feel cured."

Pamela's story is like that of many interstitial cystitis patients:

"I was about eighteen years old when I had my first attack. I remember it very well. I was working in New York City as a model, when I suddenly had to go to the bathroom. It was just uncontrollable. I managed to get to a ladies' room, and when I finally went, there was a lot of blood in the urine. Accordingly, I was treated for a bladder infection.

"But after that, the problem continued. I would go through bouts of increased urinary problems. I'd feel great urgency to urinate but very little would come out. There was a lot of pain involved. For the next twelve years, no matter what my symptoms were, I was treated for recurrent bladder infections. Many times urine cultures were not taken. It was always explained to me that I had a bladder infection that just repeatedly came back. And I was always prescribed pretty much the same medicine. They were large red pills which would relieve the pain and supposedly stop the infection.

"Some years were better than others. I'd have a month of pain and then many months pain-free. But then it would always come back. I found different things would set it off. If I had no sexual contact for a long time and then resumed it, the problem would recur. If I was under pressure, the symptoms would worsen. But one thing was consistent: No infection was ever found.

"Over the years I saw about ten doctors. Usually I was given antibiotics. Sometimes they changed their approach. One gynecologist performed a D and C [dilation and curettage] operation that scraped my uterus 'clean.' He said I had 'excessive infection with a lot of buildup.' It didn't make sense to me why he'd operate on my uterus to fix my bladder. But the funny thing is that I did feel better for a while. I'd believe in these aggressive treatments for a while. Then the pain would come back.

"Finally, one of my gynecologists sent me to a urologist. I'll never forget it. First thing, he wanted a urine sample. But instead of asking for it, he stuck a catheter up into my bladder. Now I was there because I had horrible pain. And he just went ahead and catheterized me. Of course, my urine turned out to be sterile. It was the most excrutiating thing anybody had ever done to me. Except he then proceeded to give me these so-called urethral dilation treatments to widen and stretch open the urethra. After he did that, the urine would just pour out of me for a while and I did seem to get better. Then the pain would come back.

"I had maybe three or four dilations, always accompanied by another dose of antibiotics. By this time, I was really getting scared. The last dilation gave me a genuine infection. I was worse off after going through more excruciating pain. I got to the point that I knew something more serious was wrong with me. I knew I wasn't being cured. I was uncomfortable so much of the time. One morning I looked into my medicine cabinet and saw rows of pills that I had been taking for years and I really felt very desperate."

You Are Not Alone

If you identify with Pamela Sue Martin, you are not alone. After her successful response to therapy in 1984, she and I appeared together on "Hour Magazine," a television talk show hosted by Gary Collins. My office received more than 20,000 letters from women around the country who said they had the same problem. One wrote, "I was ironing and listening to you talk when all of a sudden I realized you were talking about me!"

If you pay close attention, you probably will notice some hallmarks of this disease. The pain in your bladder feels worse after you urinate. It hurts both before and after you go to the bathroom. In fact, the only time you get relief is during those few moments when you are voiding.

You probably also have noticed that some foods make your symptoms worse. Perhaps you have eliminated coffee, tea, and orange juice from your diet, but you continue to have unexplainable bouts of pain.

Moreover, your doctor is as baffled as you are. She or he knows you're in pain but can't find anything to explain it. When your doctor looks into your bladder in the office with a cystoscope, an instrument that illuminates the inside of the bladder, everything appears normal. Your urine cultures turn up negative. You do not have a bacterial infection.

Finally, your doctor may tell you that the only way to cope with this chronic pain is through psychiatric help. He or she argues convincingly: It is a well-established tenet of urology that chronic, nonbacterial cystitis may be caused by emotional distress. *Campbell's Urology* (fourth edition, 1979, by J. Hartwell Harrison, M.D., Ruben F. Gittes, M.D., Alan D. Perlmutter, M.D., Thomas A. Stamey, M.D., and Patrick C. Walsh, M.D.), a textbook memorized by every resident in training, says it quite plainly:

"Interstitial cystitis—a disease that is taunting in its evasion of being understood—may represent the end stage of a bladder that has been made irritable by emotional disturbance."

The text then goes on to tell the story of a twenty-nine-year-old woman whose "bladder had come to serve as a pathway for the discharge of unconscious hatreds." This hatred, it says, "combined with a bladder infection during puberty to set up a vicious sequence of hate, repression of this hostile emotion, enuresis [bed-wetting] as an expression of the hatred, superimposed infection, and inflammation, all of which apparently culminated in chronic interstitial cystitis."

This was the first disease I had ever heard about in which the mind could cause an organ to burn, ulcerate, and shrink. It was the first psychiatric disease that could mysteriously cause tissue to scar. So I raised one of my "buts": But you must be telling us that women have incredibly powerful minds if we can cause our bladders to shrink. Are you giving us all that credit?

Don't Let Them Tell You It's All in Your Head

As an open-minded woman, you feel perhaps there may be some emotional problem at the root of your bladder pain. After all, you do seem to cry easily in recent months. The constant pain has had an effect on your personality. No one has a perfect childhood or nontraumatized life. So you go into therapy.

After six months, however, it starts to become clear that while you do have some problems to work through, the problems are not causing the real and genuine pain you feel before and after you urinate. Your therapist, too, agrees that you are a victim of real and not imaginary pain. But she can't help you eliminate the pain. She can only help you cope with it.

If you, as a reader, recognize this as the story of your life, then I would like to assure you that *you don't have a psychiatric disorder. You are not crazy. Your childhood mishaps have nothing to do with the constant pain you are coping with every day of your life.*

Rather, you have the devastating disease called interstitial cystitis. It is one of the least understood and most underdiagnosed diseases in modern urology. Most practitioners are under the impression that interstitial cystitis is rare. But in actuality, the failure to suspect interstitial cystitis is why so many of you are not diagnosed as having this disease.

Twigs in the Bladder

Interstitial cystitis is not new. The problem was first described by a French physician in 1836. He saw so-called ulcers on the floor of the bladder which would rupture.

The disease was again described and popularized in 1914 by Guy Hunner, a Baltimore gynecologist. He reported that he was finding a rare type of bladder ulcer in women. The back wall of the bladder was congested with blood vessels, he said, that appeared to mingle and then split up into "numerous twigs." An ulcer was frequently noted. This condition became known as *Hunner's ulcer*. Hunner did not know what caused the "twigs" but he did note that many of his patients had scarlet fever, an association which, as we'll see later, turned out to be important.

Other physicians found these "ulcers" and, in listening to their patients agonize about the pain, developed various treatments. One urologist, for example, put sandalwood oil directly into women's bladders in an attempt to keep urine from burning the tissue. Other palliatives were devised and tried but interstitial cystitis was deemed incurable. In worse cases, women had their bladders surgically removed.

Insterstitial Cystitis Defined

Over the years, physicians began to refer to Hunner's ulcer as interstitial cystitis, a more general name. "Hunner's ulcer," meanwhile, turned out to be a somewhat misleading term. Hunner saw true ulcers because his patients were suffering from an advanced stage of disease brought on most likely, we can speculate in hindsight, by streptococcal bacteria. After the advent of antibiotics in the 1940s, strep infections were largely arrested before they could damage bladder tissue and lead to interstitial cystitis. Unfortunately, physicians were taught to look for an ulcer in making a diagnosis. When they examined the bladders of women with the symptoms described by Pamela Sue Martin and others, they could not see any ulcers. Thus they failed to make the diagnosis of interstitial cystitis.

But it was also not clear that interstitial cystitis is a progressive disease, going from microscopic ulceration to a shrunken, scarred bladder. It has a continuum of stages. It has not one but many clinical manifestations. Thus today you do not have to have an end-stage bladder that holds only a half cup of urine to be finally diagnosed as having this disease. Your symptoms do not have to be so obvious that even an elevator operator could diagnose your case.

First, it is important for you to know that interstitial cystitis is not the same disease as common cystitis. There is a world of difference.

Common cystitis is an episodic inflammation of the urinary bladder caused by bacterial infection. When bacteria get into the bladder and cannot get out, they multiply and thrive in wet, warm urine. Pain is caused when bacteria attack your bladder lining, causing superficial erosion of the lining. Urine then comes into contact with sensitive tissues, setting up sensations of burning, frequency, and pressure. It hurts when you urinate.

Such bacterial infections respond to short-term antibiotic therapy. Antibiotics work by different mechanisms. Some are like detergents—they lower the surface tension on bacteria, causing the organisms to rupture and die. Others inhibit protein synthesis in the bacteria, which prevents them from multiplying rapidly.

Interstitial cystitis, on the other hand, has nothing directly to do with bacteria. It is a chronic condition caused by an inflammation of the space (called the *interstice* or *interstitium*) between the bladder lining and the bladder muscle. It is induced by a variety of agents, but bacteria generally are not present in the bladders of its victims.

However, and this is an important point, the majority of people who get interstitial cystitis have had earlier bouts in their lives with bacterial-induced cystitis. The bacteria seem to presensitize the bladder before the numerous agents we call *promoters* start the ulcerative process.

And what are those agents? We're only just beginning to find out. In my research with more than 400 interstitial cystitis patients—the largest group of such patients ever studied—I have identified several factors and cofactors that promote the disease. These include certain drugs, hormones, and a virus. I am certain there are others we have not yet identified.

The agents are different, creating different damage to cells, until they funnel into a common process: interstitial cystitis. That is, interstitial cystitis is not one disease but many, with multiple causes.

In my work with interstitial cystitis, I have become convinced that it is an environmental disease. When presensitized people come into contact with one or more environmental factors, the disease process can begin. It involves, as we shall see later on, a slow destruction of bladder tissue by urine. The immune system may try to cope with this destruction by making adaptations to bladder tissue. It is as if the body is trying to heal itself but is thwarted by a constant attack—that of urine on injured tissue.

Interstitial cystitis is progressive and exhibits a wide range of disease manifestations. In its earliest stages, frequency without bacterial infection may be all that is noted. It usually starts out as a mild condition, in which the bladder's protective inner lining becomes inactivated.

In severe cases, the bladder is ulcerated and scarred. It literally shrinks and may hold only one to two ounces of urine. In every case of interstitial cystitis, sensitive tissue is continuously exposed to an acid burn from urine. As a result, it is painful to hold urine.

In fact, as noted, the only time an interstitial cystitis patient feels relief is when she voids. During those moments, the capillaries that filter the contents of urine have no blood flow. Filtration therefore stops. But when she finishes voiding, the vessels quickly refill, causing increased filtration of acid and other elements in urine. Pain resumes.

Interstitial Cystitis Around the World

As time went on, many physicians from around the world began to notice that interstitial cystitis does not occur with the same incidence in every country. In England, for example, it has been found in one of every 660 outpatients with cystitis. In Scandinavia, it has been identified in one in 350 such patients. In the United States, some physicians believe that one in 20 cystitis sufferers is a victim of interstitial cystitis.

It seems to be more prevalent in the United States. Is there perhaps some explanation for the higher incidence? Why do the women in England develop less interstitial cystitis than women in Sweden or the United States?

One reason has to do with underdiagnosis. In England, for example, women are not thought to have the disease until their bladders shrink to half of normal capacity.

If interstitial cystitis is an environmental disease, such variations in incidence are to be expected. Women in Europe are exposed to different drugs, pollution factors, and diets from American women. These differences, I believe, explain the different rates of interstitial cystitis occurrence around the world.

Why Are So Many Cases Misdiagnosed?

Why are so many cases (perhaps yours) of interstitial cystitis overlooked or misdiagnosed? Why do some physicians believe it is a very rare disease? The answer is complex and reflects the dynamic nature of medical knowledge itself.

Interstitial cystitis is a particularly enigmatic disease. Because it was first described in detail by a gynecologist, many physicians to this day are under the false impression that only women can develop interstitial cystitis. But men get it, too. They tend to be diagnosed as having a bacterial prostatitis or nonspecific urethritis, vague-sounding conditions about which very little is known. In my experience, many men thus diagnosed actually have interstitial cystitis. If you think it is difficult to get properly diagnosed when you are female, you should consider what it is like for men with this disease. Many are given unnecessary prostatectomies (as their female counterparts are given unnecessary hysterectomies) as a way of treating the symptoms of lower pelvic pain.

Because interstitial cystitis has many causes, which funnel into common symptoms in both men and women, medical investigators have been confounded in their attempts to explain the disease. Also, much of the medical detective work today that is leading to treatments for interstitial cystitis is based on very recent medical findings. The biochemical aspects of this disease are on the forefront of the field of biochemistry itself.

Many doctors have seen only one "classic" case in their medical careers and are simply unaware that the disease widely exists. By looking for Hunner's ulcer, they miss other signs that would lead to a diagnosis. Some physicians are aware of interstitial cystitis but think it is a hopeless problem. Some, in fact, regard interstitial cystitis as a disease worse than cancer. At least there are well-established approaches and methods for treating cancer; the doctor knows what to do. But there are not yet widely agreed upon treatments for interstitial cystitis among the nation's urologists. Underdiagnosis has made it a rare, orphan disease.

Hence some physicians, when they suspect you have interstitial cystitis, might opt not to tell you. They believe they can't do anything; they don't know of any treatment that works. They think that you have an incurable disease, and that if you knew, you'd get more upset than you already are.

Here is where the importance of knowing how to be a patient comes in (see Chapter Four). If you have this chronic disease, you know how much pain there is. You know how easy it is for you to cry and become emotional about the disease. You know that the pain sometimes really does drive you "crazy." To many doctors this is proof that you are suffering from a psychiatric disorder. You act unbalanced. Your fixation on your bladder, he says, is causing it to shrink so that it may ultimately have to be removed.

You may be blubbering all over his desk, and he is a caring physician and feels helpless. So he does what any gallant gentleman does to help a lady in distress. He offers the best help he can, which is psychological counseling. He wants to help you learn to cope with the pain and look into your soul for the reason you hurt. You are referred to a psychiatrist.

Barbara's Story

In recent years, the research that several others and I have done has confirmed my suspicions that interstitial cystitis is not psychiatric. I began to suspect that the emperor had no clothes. It just did not make sense.

This became apparent when Barbara came to see me in 1980, the first year of my private practice. Her arrival marked for me the beginning of a great adventure in urology. Together we embarked on an investigation that was to be full of mysteries and surprises.

It is my habit to open the door to my waiting room and personally invite each patient into my office. It is my environment and I like to invite people in just the way I invite them into my home after opening the front door of the house.

I was immediately struck by the way Barbara walked. I still like to exercise my observational skills when meeting patients. She was dressed in a loose empire waist dress and flats and her hair seemed rigid, as if she had pushed it stiffly into place. Her face was drawn.

Before standing up, she looked at me with a quick, almost furtive glance, which seemed to say, "I'm scared and suspicious of you. You probably won't believe what I say."

She stood up painfully and began to walk. Her legs were apart and she took small, slow, careful steps to avoid jarring her body. It was what I have come to call the "classic interstitial cystitis walk." In my office, she gripped the arms of the chair and lowered herself, again slowly, into the seat. Then she shifted her weight off her pelvis.

I asked her what I could do to help. Barbara did not, could not, look me in the face. This was a pattern I was to see many times in people with this disease. She refused to meet my eyes out of a fear that I would not believe her story. Like many interstitial cystitis patients, Barbara had been told there was nothing really wrong with her.

The facts of her story were tragic. She recounted them recently, going over some of the things she told me when we met: "I began having urinary problems six years ago, when I was twenty-eight years old. It began with urine retention for no reason anyone could figure out. I was dilated two or three times a week. They couldn't find a cause for my problem. Although I started out with bladder infections, later they could not find infections. It was just bladder pain that continued for four to five years.

"I reached the point where the pain was so great I began to go to other doctors. I was told I had kidney problems. I was told I'd be on dialysis by the time I was forty. The pain increased and I was given antibiotics. I was maintained on antibiotics for years. The sulfa drugs made me shaky and the other antibiotics made me tired all the time. No one warned me of the side effects. My energy was draining and draining. I was working as a literary agent in New York and was always exhausted.

"Then I developed lower back problems. They seemed to be related to the urinary retention. I went in and out of emergency wards for dilation, back traction, and new regimes of antibiotics.

"I knew I could not maintain my life the way it was. At thirty-three, I left New York for California, believing inside of me that I would not live long. Every day, every night I was frightened and no one could give me a reason for my pain and fear.

"The search for doctors who could help continued. My pain increased and my back problems worsened. I'd suddenly be unable to walk, spend two weeks in the hospital and six months recovering. I found urologists mostly to be plumbers. They described the machinery, how it works, and told me everything in my body worked fine. One doctor scraped the inside of my bladder and trigone. It was called a curettage, supposedly kind of like a D and C of the bladder. It made me much worse.

"I was always left with the feeling that I had somehow done something wrong to my body. I was somehow responsible for creating the mysterious pain. This implication, that the pain was not there, is, for me, the hardest part. It eroded my spirit.

Imagine a woman in pain whom no one has ever believed! She was trying to cope but the pain was winning. Barbara had been to fifteen doctors (about average for women with this problem) complaining of unremitting lower pelvic pain. She was occasionally told she had pelvic inflammatory disease, or PID.

In reality, the pain of PID cannot match up to the pain of interstitial cystitis. I have had a child and occasionally experience menstrual cramps so I know what pelvic pain can feel like. But with interstitial cystitis, there is a continuous acid burn of the tissue on top of the cramping.

As Barbara told her story that day in my office, she began to weep. Her emotional pain predominated her physical pain. And as she spoke, I realized why other physicians probably had had a hard time listening to her: hardly any facts were being related; it was all emotion.

After she finished, I said, "I think I know what's wrong with you." Barbara looked stunned. It was the first time any physician had said that. As she calmed down, I asked her questions.

Does it hurt before, during, or after you urinate? She had not thought to pay attention before but, yes, it only stopped hurting when she voided.

Are you very meticulous and obsessive about neatness? Do you make lists? This question was prompted by my then recent medical training, which taught me that interstitial cystitis patients are so-called Type A personalities. Today I think these personality traits are irrelevant to the disease. Anyway, Barbara's answer was affirmative; she was Type A.

Have cultures been done on your urine? She answered, "Very few." Nevertheless, Barbara was repeatedly prescribed antibiotics to combat infections. I found this interesting. I never give antibiotics without first getting a urine sample for culturing. As time went on, Barbara said, she began to notice that the antibiotics made her symptoms worse. She had to urinate more and more often.

Did you try psychotherapy? Yes, and after several years, she found she could handle the pain better. But the pain did not lessen.

The GAG Layer

To understand what happened to Barbara's bladder and perhaps to yours, you need to visualize how a healthy bladder works. On the bladder surface there is a protective layer that is secreted, like mucus, from the cells that make up the bladder lining. Scientifically speaking, this secretion is made of sulfated glycosaminoglycans, but from now on we'll simply call it your GAG layer.

The GAG layer, a fouling barrier, is your first line of protection against anything that enters your bladder. Urine contains many toxic elements that your body has excreted. The GAG layer repels them. It is like a moisturizer that keeps harmful elements from interacting with tissue.

Perhaps most importantly, the GAG layer is impervious to acids and toxins found in urine. It is believed that by binding to underlying cells, the GAG layer creates an electrically neutral barrier to urine. Specifically, the GAG layer is designed to prevent protons—electrically positive-charged elements in urine—from binding to the surface of the underlying tissue. Without a GAG layer, the underlying bladder tissue cells would readily interact with electrically charged chemicals in your urine. A tiny electric current would be established across the cellular membranes—protons would flow from urine into the unprotected cells and you would feel "electric shocks."

Furthermore, your GAG layer is the primary antibacterial defense mechanism of the bladder. When bacteria enter a normal bladder under normal circumstances, the layer prevents them from adhering to the interior tissue. The bacteria are soon washed away and no harm is done. But if bacteria remain in the bladder, they begin to colonize. Growing bacteria secrete enzymes that help them adhere to tissue. The more bacteria, the more enzymes. Eventually, the GAG layer is eroded. Bacteria begin to adhere to underlying bladder cells.

When this protective layer is damaged, urine gains access to tissue below. This can have several effects. Cell membranes begin to leak. Capillaries are exposed to urine. And nerve networks in the bladder are inappropriately triggered. Between epithelial cells (the cells of the bladder lining) there are branches of sensory nerves that are connected to the sympathetic nervous system. When a normal bladder is half full, the GAG layer is slightly stretched, which allows ions or chemicals in urine to leak across the barrier and tickle or excite these nerves below. This gives rise to the signal to void. But in a damaged bladder, ions in much smaller volumes of urine get through the barrier. You feel burning, pressure, cramping, frequency, and pain—the hallmarks of cystitis.

In a study of 300 patients with interstitial cystitis, I found that more than 95 percent of them had a history of at least one bacteria-proven bladder infection. This led me to speculate that when a healthy GAG layer is damaged—particularly by recurrent bacterial infections—it may change, or mutate. The affected bladder may later be more susceptible to other chemicals and be ineffective at deflecting them from the tissue. Once your GAG layer is compromised, your chances of developing abnormal tissue in response to urinary toxins are higher than if your bladder was never modified.

As previously stated, there are many agents—certain drugs, hormones, pesticides, a virus and so on—that may serve as promoters of interstitial cystitis. In Hunner's day, scarlet fever was such an agent. If you have interstitial cystitis, you have probably been exposed to something that has compromised your GAG layer. Thus it is important to recall any circumstances surrounding the onset of your disease.

The onset of interstitial cystitis can be insidious and slow, but it can also be sudden and traumatic. Diane, for example, went to a friend's wedding and began the two-hour drive home with a full bladder. She had to urinate but decided to hold it in since she was "almost home." She had had a few bladder infections in her life but noticed nothing unusual. Once home, she ran to the bathroom and sat down to void. At that moment, she developed tremendous pain. And from that moment forward, she never voided normally again. Her onset was related to the way she overdistended her bladder by holding in urine for so long. Upon questioning, it became clear that her bladder was not normal, as she came to realize she had been having symptoms of frequency and mild burning for quite some time. But she had paid them no heed until the wedding episode precipitated her problem and made her look into it.

Symptoms and Concepts

As I listened to Diane and then to hundreds of other women with interstitial cystitis, I slowly pieced together different aspects of this enigmatic disease. Each patient's story contained clues about what causes interstitial cystitis and clues to developing treatments that work. Deciphering the meaning of various symptoms has led to developing fundamental concepts of the disease.

Symptom: Acid Foods Make Me Feel Worse

One of the first things I asked patients in those early days of my practice was simply, "What makes you feel better or worse?" Frequently, one answer was, "Acid foods make me feel terrible."

"I discovered I couldn't drink orange juice, grapefruit juice, or other acid drinks without increasing the burning and pain," said Paula, an Orange County housewife who was immobilized for several years with interstitial cystitis. "Wine was the worst. My bladder would start to hurt almost instantly."

Esther said she had been taking vitamin C by the handfuls. "Before I'd have breakfast I'd feel better. An hour later I'd be uncomfortable. I also lived on grapefruit and toast for breakfast and drink cranberry juice all day long. I thought I was doing my body all sorts of good."

So in looking for a common element, I decided to look at how acids might be involved with bladder pain. The simplest way to do this involved testing the pH of urine voided by my patients.

The symbol *pH* is used to describe the acidity or alkalinity of a solution. Acid solutions have a pH measuring from 0 to 7. Alkaline solutions have a pH of 7 to 14. A neutral solution, which is neither acid nor alkaline, has a pH of 7. Acids, by definition, are solutions that donate positively charged hydrogen ions (called protons). Alkaline bases, by definition, are solutions that accept protons.

At first, I suspected I would find that my patients would have very acid urine. After all, they complained of acidlike burns in the bladder. When they ate acid foods, their symptoms worsened. Was acid urine to blame?

Surprisingly, I found the opposite: My patients all had very alkaline urine! Now, I had been taught that alkaline urine is not abnormal. They were merely called "alkaline tides" and were supposedly related to dietary influence.

But this didn't make sense. I was measuring alkaline urine in patients who hadn't eaten for twelve hours. When you don't eat for that long, your urine becomes acid. These patients should have been, to use the medical term, acidotic. I tested urines at different times of the day and consistently saw alkaline urine in association with severe pain, burning, and frequency. It became clear to me that the high pH of their urine was not related to diet.

To prove it, I had patients' husbands eat exactly the same diet as their wives and then I recorded their urinary pH. The husbands' pH hardly ever went above 5.5, which is normal for most urine samples. Yet the wives, with the same diet and fluid intake, showed pHs of 7.5, with marked symptoms of pain and burning.

I then asked myself: Is the urine in their kidneys alkaline or is it just urine in the bladder that has an elevated pH? Logically, if alkaline urine correlated with what you ate, the urine in the kidneys should show it.

I ran a very simple experiment in the operating room. While patients were anesthetized, I ran catheters up their ureters to get urine samples from the kidneys. Sure enough, the urinary pH in the kidneys was in the normal pH range of 5.5. Urine in the bladder was somehow undergoing significant pH changes. Since the bladder serves as a reservoir for fluids, there would be plenty of time for a chemical change to occur there.

Concept: How Leaky Cell Membranes Contribute to Pain

This discovery of pH changes was the first breakthrough in solving the mystery. It pinpointed that interstitial cystitis involved the chemistry of the bladder lining. The pH changes were not irrelevant. Rather they were a clue to explaining the disease process.

I reasoned there must be an ion exchange occurring on the bladder surface. Positive charges found in normally acid urine were disappearing! Instead, the urine was showing excess negative charges, resulting in an alkaline urine. What could account for this basic chemical change?

I began to think about cells. Cells are fundamentally alkaline. They contain high levels of bicarbonate, which gives them an alkaline pH (see illustration, below).

If cells were leaking, two things could happen. First, the cells would lose bicarbonate as negative charges in the cells flow out toward the positive charges in the urine (positive and negative charges attract one another). That would explain how the urine became alkaline. Second, positive charges in urine would start flowing toward negative charges in the cells. Urine would enter the leaking cells. And it would burn.

At that point, I remembered what I had been taught about burn patients. They lose massive amounts of bicarbonate, an alkaline salt. In fact, one of the most critical aspects of treating burn patients is to give them lots of sodium bicarbonate (a sodium alkaline salt) to arrest the cellular leakage of bicarbonate.

It occurred to me that my patients were describing the identical problem. If you drip acid on your arm, you will get a burn and a loss of bicarbonate. If you keep acid urine on your injured bladder, you will experience burning and loss of bicarbonate. The pH readings proved it.

Suddenly I knew the direction to take. By postulating interstitial cystitis as a "leaky cell membrane" disease, I could look for factors that would cause the leak to occur. And I could try to find ways to stop the leak.

Clearly, healthy bladders with intact GAG layers do not leak. Urine, with all its toxic substances and high acidity, does not burn or injure a normal bladder. But if you constantly put urine directly on skin that has no protective GAG layer, you will get a burn. Men and women who are incontinent develop terrible burns in their genital area on the skin; their skin takes on the texture of nonpliable leather.

I developed a model of a leaky urothelial cell, that is one that has lost its GAG layer protection (see illustration). When the GAG layer is lost, the charges from urine can affect the exposed bladder membrane. The cells, in turn, exchange negative charges for the positive ones in urine. A balance is achieved.

As I developed this model, a patient one day told me she was taking baking soda for her symptoms and found it helpful. Instead of dismissing this as irrelevant, I wondered how that could possibly help.

Baking soda is alkaline. It would make the urine in the kidney less acid, I reasoned. In turn, urine reaching the bladder would be less acid and therefore less highly charged.

This turns out to be beneficial for the person with leaky cell membranes. When cells leak, they lose sodium and gain hydrogen. It is as if the cell pumps one element in and another out. When urine pH is altered with baking soda, the pump mechanism is reversed. The cells begin to regain sodium bicarbonate and to lose hydrogen ions (protons). This restores the normal alkaline balance of the cells.

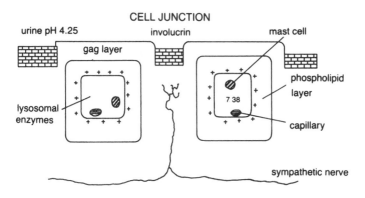

Figure 2-1, Leaky Urothelial Cell

Another patient said her symptoms were relieved by pyridium but not by urised, both bladder anesthetic agents. I looked up urised and discovered it would only work in an acid medium. Since my patients' urine was not acid, the medication urised naturally did not work, and neither did it turn their urine blue, as it does for people whose urine is acid. Pyridium, on the other hand, is not related to pH. It, by the way, turns urine orange by releasing mahogany dye. One patient said she felt like an Easter bunny: She dyed all her underwear red or blue depending on which medicine she was taking.

Symptom: Urinary Frequency

About this time I started asking patients to describe their pain in more detail. What kind of pressure feeling is it? Many then said it felt like spasms.

"You don't sleep at night," said Pam. "You lie there looking at the ceiling and say, 'Why me?' The pain is constant. You feel like you've swallowed a strep throat and it's lodged in your bladder."

This was puzzling. Urologic investigations had shown that the smooth bladder muscle, the detrusor, does not actually spasm. But there was no denying that patients were describing real cramps, even to the extent of comparing them to the cramps of childbirth.

It made me think. If you keep putting acid on a wound, it eats away at tissue and gets right down to the bone. If the urine is burning bladder tissue, the bladder would "want" to rid itself of urine as quickly as possible. It makes sense that bladder spasms are a protective response of the body, to keep its surface from being burned further. If you keep washing the acid away, you may contain the burn to a lesser level. Thus the symptom of urinary frequency became one of the earliest indicators that the process of interstitial cystitis had begun.

I also reexamined what I'd been taught about diagnosing this disease. One of the hallmarks of the disease is a shrunken, shriveled bladder. Thinking again of burns, I realized that when the skin forms a scar, the skin contracts—plastic reconstructive surgery is based on concepts of how to release scar tissue and regain mobility and flexibility.

A bladder with end-stage interstitial cystitis would shrink as if with scar tissue. As the burning continued, the bladder would no longer expand and contract normally. I remembered Hunner's ulcers. Now it was clear to me why the disease had been classified as ulcerative. Urine is indeed ulcerating and could burn away the very lining of the bladder.

Concept: Urethritis as an Early Sign

I realized that the ability to diagnose their disease only at this very late, ulcerative, stage was little help to my patients. I needed to find the earliest sign of the disease. I pulled charts on patients I had diagnosed as having "urethritis." The term *urethritis,* defined as inflammation of the urethra, has no real meaning, but it was the term available at the time.

I called some of those patients months after having seen them to ask, "How are you doing? Do you still have your symptoms?" They were surprised to hear from me but, yes, the symptoms were continuing. "I have to urinate every hour," said Cindy. "It feels like pressure in my urethra, a kind of irritation down there. It isn't getting any better."

I began to suspect that urethritis could be the beginnings of interstitial cystitis. Upon reexamination, these women had nothing wrong with their urethras. There was no inflammation and no redness. I wondered if something could be happening in the bladder that was causing the external sphincter in the urethra to go into spasm. This would make their symptom a referral pain; that is, pain that originates in one place but is felt in another. Was the urethra being blamed for a problem in the bladder? At the time, there was no known nerve pathway that could account for this kind of referral pain. (The pathway was later found. See page 78.)

Symptoms: Antibiotics Make It Worse

By asking patients, "What makes you feel worse?" another pattern emerged.

"I had dozens of attacks," said Linda. "My doctor was great about it. I'd just call him and tell him I had another infection and he'd renew my prescription for an antibiotic. We didn't bother to do urine cultures because we knew I was just one of those women who got cystitis a lot.

"But after a while, I noticed that the antibiotics weren't working. My symptoms wouldn't go away in a couple of days. In fact, sometimes they got worse. We tried several antibiotics but I kept getting worse."

Before long, more than thirty patients told me, separately and without any coaching, that their symptoms got worse when they took antibiotics. But not just any antibiotics but three particular drugs: nitrofurantoin, tetracycline, and erythromycin.

These patients' past urinalysis reports showed marked elevation of urinary pH but no bacteria growth in the urine culture. There seemed to be no explanation for their urinary symptoms.

But a pattern seemed to be emerging.

When one patient informed me that her urine smelled like "a dead mouse" just before a bad attack, I pulled the charts on past patients and realized that the patients who were coming back to me because of chronic urethritis were the very ones for whom I had prescribed nitrofurantoin. These were patients I may have chastised for wearing tight jeans, saying, "You're bringing the urethritis on yourself by causing irritation to your urethra."

But maybe they were telling me something else, something significant. I had given them antibiotics three or four months at a time, but the treatment I had been taught to give in residency training was not working for these patients. They were not responding; in fact, the patients' symptoms had changed for the worse: Now they felt pain and burning all the time, except when urinating. Their stories were sounding exactly like interstitial cystitis. It suddenly felt more like a murder mystery than a simple *medical* mystery. Were doctors doing in their own patients?

Concept: Antibiotic-Related Interstitial Cystitis

Like other urologists, I had been taught that so-called chronic antibiotic suppressive therapy was the proper way to treat women complaining of repeated urinary tract infections. In this therapy, the patient takes antibiotics every day for three to four months. The rationale? Something is chronically inducing her infections, so you should simply knock out the bacteria before they take hold.

There are several problems with this concept. As discussed in Chapter One, there is usually a common sense cause for repeated urinary infections. When something obstructs the normal flow of urine, bacteria have greater opportunity to grow in the bladder. Lower back problems are also often a reason for cystitis, as will be discussed. In my opinion, the only time it makes sense to take antibiotics for long periods is when conditions such as a chronic kidney infection or bladder paralysis are present.

Another question was whether or not bacteria were present when these medications were taken. Many patients told me they did not give urine cultures before taking long cycles of antibiotics.

What if they had not had bacteria in their urine? What if they were taking antibiotics in the absence of infection? What if their symptoms—frequency, burning, pain—were *not* caused by bacteria?

I began to think about how antibiotics work. There are two main mechanisms. Bacteriocidal drugs—ampicillin, penicillin, and sulfa drugs—work by killing bacteria outright. Other antibiotics attack the bacterial membrane. They invade the outer membranes of bacteria and cause them to "leak to death." These *bacteriostatic* drugs include nitrofurantoin, tetracycline, and erythromycin.

Now there was a key to the mystery. Could it be that antibiotics—in the absence of bacteria—end up attacking what's available, namely bladder tissue? Remember: The bladder is a reservoir. An antibiotic excreted in urine that is not put to work killing bacteria would remain biologically active in the bladder. In addition, some patients could have metabolic difficulties in digesting or breaking down the drug normally. As a result, *a different or more toxic form of the antibiotic might be excreted in urine*.

There are scientific papers suggesting that this may be the case. When bacteria invade the bladder, they excrete an enzyme that yields a good supply of *ammonium ions,* a breakdown product of ammonia. Bacteria then use the ammonium ions to help them adhere to the bladder surface. An ammonium ion works by binding to a portion of the GAG molecule and impairing the molecule's ability to repel charges.

You can think of the GAG layer as being like a perimeter alarm. Its job is to keep out intruders, such as electrically charged chemicals in urine. By producing ammonium ions, bacteria inactivate the perimeter alarm. Intruders cross into unprotected cells of the bladder. The GAG layer is weakened by bacteria. It is simply inactivated.

The antibiotics tetracycline and erythromycin and nitrofurantoin (which is an antiseptic or detergent) work by inactivating the protective coat (which is much like a GAG layer) around individual bacteria. When the drugs reach a bladder that contains bacteria, they selectively target the bacteria and make them leak to death.

As it turns out, nitrofurantoin contains ammonium ions. If it were excreted into a bladder with no bacteria present, it could conceivably interact with a presensitized GAG layer and inactivate the perimeter alarm. Symptoms of burning and pain would thus accompany taking the drug.

Once a GAG perimeter is altered by bacteria (particularly by repeated infections), it may become easier for agents that are not as potent as bacteria to breach the perimeter. There are weak links in the fence.

Thus the perimeter alarm is presensitized. Although it functions, it no longer functions well. And, continuously assaulted, the perimeter eventually breaks down and loses resistance. Perhaps this is why chronic antibiotic therapy in the absence of infection seems to be a common link among patients with interstitial cystitis.

It might also explain why some patients noticed their urine smelled like a dead mouse. Something—perhaps a metabolic problem in breaking down proteins—could be producing excessive ammonium ions in urine. The result is a noxious smell, hence the graphic description.

The antibiotics associated with interstitial cystitis are not always prescribed for bladder infections. Many women take these drugs for acne or bronchitis. In cream form, they can be absorbed into the body in large amounts. Thus, some patients may later develop interstitial cystitis without ever having had cystitis. Antibiotic-related interstitial cystitis is largely an American version of the disease. In certain European countries, for example, nitrofurantoin, erythromycin, and tetracycline are not generally prescribed by physicians. This may help explain the relatively high incidence of interstitial cystitis in the United States, where these drugs are given routinely for the presumptive diagnosis of infection.

Please understand me: Antibiotics are not bad for you if you have a case of true bacterial cystitis. In that case, the antibiotic does what it is designed to do—inactivates the bacteria.

But if you insist that your doctor give you an antibiotic over the telephone without an exam every time your cystitis "flares up," or you get a cough or flu attack, you may be inviting more pain and suffering upon yourself. If the physician prescribes medication without taking a urine culture first to prove there is bacteria in your urine, you are asking for trouble.

Incidentally, to date there has never been a satisfactory animal model for interstitial cystitis. The complex of symptoms and the disease, however, are real. One difficulty with the studies that have been done is that they use animal bladders that have not been presensitized by a previous bacterial infection. In addition, one virus implicated in the disease cannot be introduced into rats, mice, or rabbits. Without laying this basis, as well as introducing important cofactors in the disease process, the results of research on animals have been confused and conflicting.

Finally, it is important that urologists discard the notion that women are "loaded" with bacteria and fated to get recurrent urinary tract infections. It is this bias, I believe, that leads to the improper use of antibiotics in treating the symptoms of cystitis.

More Symptoms

CHOCOLATE AND OTHER FOODS

While patients said acid foods worsened their symptoms, other foods were also singled out.

"I get really bad when I eat chocolate," said one.

"Champagne and red wine destroy me," said another.

"If I eat Mexican food, the burn really increases," said another. One Chinese woman told me ruefully that she could not tolerate soy sauce.

Soon I found myself sitting with a list of foods. What common element did they have? How could they be implicated with bladder function?

The list multiplied like rabbits. It soon included carbonated drinks, coffee, cheese, nuts, bananas, yogurt, avocado, and raisins.

THE ELECTRIC SHOCK SYNDROME

Meanwhile, many patients reported they felt a bizarre sensation in the bladder. "The pain is somewhat like a cramp," said Georgianne, "with a little electric shock in it. Zit! It keeps getting you every ten to fifteen seconds. It goes on all day long until you become debilitated and exhausted by the pain."

These "electric shocks" were somewhat different from the chemical burn most patients felt. The sensations were sharp, tingling, as if they involved nerves.

Such symptoms, interestingly, were exacerbated by stress. "I really notice it when I'm under pressure," said Nancy. "The more stress at work or home, the more my bladder hurts."

OTHER DRUGS INTENSIFYING DISCOMFORT

Other patients said certain medications made them much worse. These included several over-the-counter cold medicines and some long-lasting cough drops.

Louise was addicted to diet pills even though she had bladder attacks every time she took amphetamines. Like many compulsive dieters, she denied she might be hurting herself with so many diet pills. And for Louise, the correlation between the pills and her bladder was unmistakable. She chose to ignore it for a year and then checked herself into a drug therapy program. When free of the diet pills, her symptoms abated.

Mary asked me why her symptoms always flared up when she had dental work done. "Are my teeth related to my bladder?" she asked. I investigated the drugs used by dentists, Xylocaine (the trademark for Lignocaine) with adrenaline. How might they fit the puzzle?

There were also some patients who found that the antidepressant Elavil (amitriptyline), prescribed by their psychiatrists, really helped quell their symptoms. "The first time I took it," said Betty, "it felt like the fire was stomped out. But it was too strong to take at the dosages given me so I cut my pills way down and used only a small amount every night."

PAINFUL INTERCOURSE

A most debilitating symptom for many of my patients is painful intercourse. There are sharp pains in the vagina upon penetration which go away (temporarily) only if an orgasm is achieved.

"It is ruining my marriage," said Astrid. "My husband thinks I'm making it up and just want an excuse not to sleep with him. But the pain is terrible. It hurts and it doesn't go away with time. I've tried relaxing, different lubricants, even aspirin before sex. It just plain hurts."

Concept: How Nerve System Chemicals Can Trigger Bladder Pain

About the time I was trying to make sense of all these various symptoms, new scientific findings were published about an important chemical component of the nervous system. Very powerful chemicals previously identified in the brain (the neurotransmitters acetylcholine, norepinephrine, and serotonin) were found to exist—to everyone's surprise—in the gut and bladder.

Reports pointed out that these chemicals are carried along nerves that go from the brain, to the heart, to the gut, to the bladder and urethra, and finally to the tip of the penis or its feminine counterpart, the clitoris. It is an integrated system.

These nerves comprise a kind of network to be used in the body's "fight or flight" response. When an animal is stressed, these nerves "fire" their special chemicals more rapidly to help the animal escape (flight) or otherwise deal with the stressful stimulus (fight). The same is true in humans.

In bladder tissue, the nerves were found throughout the lamina propria, the bladder's very thin, smooth muscle layer in the interstitium. Previously, this layer was thought to have no function.

Since these nerves are there, I thought, what could affect their function? I had little training in nutrition but soon found that some foods contain these same powerful chemicals. These chemicals are later excreted in urine.

It was thus I discovered that foods on the list compiled by patients all contained tryptophan, tyramine, and tyrosine. In the body, these compounds stimulate the synthesis of serotonin and noradrenaline, both neurotransmitters used along this newly found system. In other words, when you eat chocolate or bananas or drink red wine, you promote the manufacture of serotonin, and a higher than usual amount of its metabolites are excreted in urine.

I searched for scientific articles on serotonin. In one study, a researcher reported cutting his finger and accidentally dropping serotonin on the wound. As a result, an enormous burn developed, and his finger swelled dramatically. There is a rare syndrome in which people produce too much serotonin. Some victims suffer itching under the arms, sore feet, hivelike sensations, and a needlelike tingling on their skins. Serotonin releases destabilized cell membranes. If a woman had a leaky perimeter alarm, an influx of ions could flow across the membrane like an electric charge. Could this produce the "electric shocks" some patients were experiencing in their bladders?

Norepinephrine and acetylcholine, the other neurotransmitters found in this nerve system, fire more rapidly along nerves when the patient is under stress, and also give rise to the symptoms of burning and cramping.

But there was another key. These neurotransmitter-conducting nerves go from the bladder through the urethra and out to the clitoris. If there was a membrane leak in the bladder stimulating transmission along these nerve routes, pain could be referred along these nerves to the next system down the road—namely the external sphincter in the urethra and the clitoris. This sounded like the needling, shooting urethral pains described by some patients. Many women had told me they had a bruised, achy feeling in the clitoris. They also said they never dared tell this symptom to a male doctor for fear he would think they were crazy.

For example, one of my patients said she told her gynecologist many years ago that her clitoris felt bruised and achy, almost throbbing with a sensation of pressure. His response was, "If it hurts, don't touch it." She said she was so shocked at being made to feel guilty for describing this observation that she never dared volunteer the symptom to another physician.

Another patient—a young woman who had been sexually active for six years and married for more than one year—said that her physician, upon hearing the symptom of clitoral pain, told her, "Oh, don't worry. You're just a nervous bride!"

But now the reason behind painful intercourse is clear. These nerves travel a route between the vagina and the base of the bladder. On one side, nerves enter the bladder's sensory region, the trigone. On the other side, they enter the vagina's sensory region, the G spot. During intercourse, the normal focal point of stimulation in the vagina is at this G spot. Now imagine there is a burning sensation in the trigone as ions stimulate the nerves of this system. The stimulation of intercourse would be like someone rubbing your sunburned back. Instead of feeling warm and tender, you feel an intensified burn, almost as if you had a third-degree sunburn in the vagina.

An orgasm, however, eradicates the pain because the nerves are temporarily inhibited. Many physicians, as well as husbands and lovers, have thought that women use interstitial cystitis to avoid sex. But in my experience, patients are deeply disturbed about the loss of sexual pleasure. They mourn the loss of pleasurable sexual intercourse.

Carolyn broke down and cried one day in my office. "Sex has always been good between my husband and me," she said. "It's just a nice thing we do together. Now I see him and he looks so sad. We lost something we valued so much. I feel bad, not for me, but for him. I see that look in his eye and I want to cry. I know he's afraid of hurting me, even when I do feel better."

As a woman, I have been deeply moved by the sexual problems faced by Carolyn and other patients. Many women are frightened of losing their marriages. Others feel they could never commit to matrimony because the pain of intercourse would prevent such intimacy.

Husbands and lovers are also deeply affected by this disease. A lover does not want to cause pain. When he cannot give sexual pleasure to his partner, he feels inadequate; he loses self-esteem and feels sexually inadequate. Thus, interstitial cystitis can change the body image and sexuality of both men and women.

Sex is possible for interstitial cystitis patients who have not completed therapy, however, with some modifications. There are many ways to express intimacy. The idea is to prevent the angle of the penis from stimulating the base of the bladder. Only certain positions accomplish this. The woman on top can lower herself onto the penis and monitor the angle herself. Or she can rest on her hands and knees as her partner enters from behind. Or he can sit on the side of the bed with the woman sitting on top of him. In this position pelvic rocking motions should not overstimulate the bladder, for the penis is against the cervix rather than the bladder.

Pain management techniques, like those taught in natural childbirth classes, work well for many patients. Peggy, for example, has her husband stroke her stomach every night at bedtime. "He uses a feather-light touch," she said, "and traces circles over my abdomen. He can feel when my bladder is tight or in spasm." According to Peggy, the technique of light stroking (called *effleurage*) relaxes her bladder. "It gives my husband a sense of really helping me," she said, "and enables me to have intercourse without bladder pain."

To help couples like Peggy and her husband, the Interstitial Cystitis Foundation offers a two-day course on sex therapy and pain management/relaxation techniques. Taught by myself and a sex therapist who has interstitial cystitis, the course shows patients how to lead full sex lives. Slow breathing and other progressive relaxation techniques, we have found, can break bladder spasms, increase sharing and trust, and make intercourse less stressful. For information on the course, see Appendix A.

Other strategies for controlling the pain also work. When I began to put my patients on a diet that restricted foods containing precursors to serotonin, their symptoms lessened. I then looked for drugs that might block serotonin's effect on membranes. I recalled the patient who told me that Elavil (amitriptylene) made her feel better. It is an antidepressant that works by blocking the uptake in membranes of serotonin, norepinephrine, and acetylcholine. This drug's blocking effect decreased the burning sensation. Only minute amounts, about 10 to 40 milligrams, eliminated most of the burn.

We soon discovered why other medications increased pain. Many cold remedies contain ephedrine, a drug that increases the production of noradrenaline and its uptake by membranes. The dentist adds adrenaline to the Xylocaine (Lignocaine) to make it last longer. And amphetamines also increase the effect of norepinephrine on membrane surfaces. This stimulates the norepinephrine-related nerves in the lamina propria, causing increased cramping.

All these symptoms now made sense in light of the brain-to-bladder chemical system of the body. With this knowledge, we could begin to treat symptoms by finding and using agents that blocked serotonin uptake and recommending that patients avoid substances that promote serotonin production.

Symptom: "Migraine" of the Bladder

Patients are very adept at describing their discomfort. The pain of interstitial cystitis has been likened to putting hot coals or sandpaper in the bladder.

But one of the most enlightening descriptions for me was: "You know, it feels like a migraine in my bladder. The pain throbs. It's as if there were a vice grip inside me and something is applying merciless pressure."

Serotonin is an agent that causes narrowing of the blood vessels. Migraine headaches are related to reduced blood flow through the small blood vessels in the brain. When there is increased serotonin available, the vessels go into spasm. This is the throbbing sensation of vascular congestion. I was struck by the fact that many patients said their migraine headaches also went away when they followed the interstitial cystitis diet restrictions! At the same time, I suspected that serotonin was not the only factor in this complex of symptoms. In examining the bladders of scores of patients, I was struck with how reddened the tissue appeared. The bladder walls were streaked with numerous blood vessels and spiraling capillaries. Normal bladders are clear and have just a few well-defined blood vessels.

I began photographing these abnormal bladders with special camera equipment (see photograph on page 84). A pattern emerged. Indeed, these were "angry" red bladders, always showing the "twigs" described by Hunner. The more I looked at them, the more they seemed to remind me of something familiar.

One day, sitting at my desk with pictures of bladders spread out in front of me, it hit me: These bladders looked like the back of the eyes of patients who have been blinded by diabetes. One of the complications of diabetes is massive capillary growth in the eye, and these bladders were marked by massive capillary growth. Some capillaries took the shape of dramatic spirals, something never seen in healthy bladders.

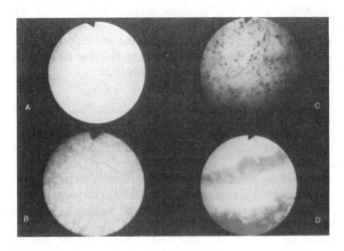

Figure 2-2, (A) A normal bladder. (B) The "angry" red bladder of interstitial cystitis. (C, D) Diverse manifestations of interstitial cystitis.

Other researchers had mentioned that there were vascular changes in the appearance of interstitial cystitis bladders. Yet no one had thought it amounted to much.

How Abnormal Capillary Growth Causes "Angry" Bladders Concept

By coincidence, at this time I read a paper on angiogenesis—a fancy word for capillary growth. Researchers at a major university had shown that capillary growth was involved in the growth of tumors. Cancerous tumors, they found, somehow encourage the proliferation of tiny capillaries, which connect the incipient tumor to nearby arteries and veins. The increased blood supply nourishes the tumor. They also found that cancer cells make a protein that promotes this capillary growth. Through special genetic engineering techniques, they are learning to make this protein in quantity for laboratory experiments.

This protein stimulates capillary growth. But if blocked, might it arrest capillary growth? I wondered.

I began to see a fuller picture of what is happening in the bladders of interstitial cystitis patients. When you cut or burn yourself, millions of tiny capillary loops are formed to seal the edges. A scab forms and later new skin grows there. But in the bladder, urine continually rips the scab from the healing site. Newly formed capillaries are continuously formed. The body is trying to heal itself, but the urine defeats it. Capillaries continue to grow unabatedly and to mature into larger vessels.

Symptoms: Joint Pains, Wheezing, Bowel Problems

As if patients with interstitial cystitis don't suffer enough, many report symptoms such as joint pains, bowel problems, fever, and asthmatic-like wheezing. Estelle's thumb always ached just before an attack of interstitial cystitis. She thought it was a sign of arthritis, even though the pain in her thumb correlated exactly with the pain in her bladder.

I began to wonder if perhaps the body's immune system was somehow involved. Many researchers over the years have suggested that interstitital cystitis may be an autoimmune disease. This means that the body has somehow made a disastrous mistake; it recognizes something in itself as being "foreign" and wages an immune system attack on its own tissue, in this case bladder tissue.

The immune system, in broad terms, involves the interplay of two agents—foreign invaders *(antigens)* and the body's own defense substances *(antibodies),* which immobilize invaders. An antigen can be a bacterium, a virus, or any number of agents from outside your body. Antibodies are proteins that recognize antigens with high specificity.

There is a highly significant test that can tell whether or not tissue from an organ has been attacked by antibodies. Called *immunofluorescence,* it literally tags the invading antigens with a fluorescent green dye. The antigens seek out antibodies (as heat-seeking missiles find a target) in tissue. If the antigen recognizes an antibody, a complex is formed and the dye fluoresces under a special light. It "sticks" to the tissue that has the antigen-antibody complex.

I wanted to know if the bladder tissue of my patients showed the presence of antibodies. Their presence would indicate that the immune system had somehow been activated. I presumed (and later proved) that normal bladder tissue does not show such activity; when tagged with the glow in the dark dye, it doesn't light up.

I sent some tissue samples from the bladders of my patients to an immunopathologist who specialized in this technique. He questioned why he should run the tests. "This is a waste of your patients' money," he said. "The bladder is not an immunologically active organ."

I insisted he run the tests on just five patients. If no activity was evident, so be it. But if antibodies showed up in the tissue, he would agree to perform this test on the biopsies of all my patients.

The tissue samples of all five patients were strikingly positive, lighting up like the glow-in-the-dark wands used by kids on Halloween. He concurred, "There's something here all right. All other bladder tissue we've seen has been totally negative." He agreed to keep investigating more patients with me.

We did 100 more tissue samples, and a pattern emerged. There were distinct categories of antibody reactions in these patients. It looked as if this was not one disease, but many. There were at least five different immunofluorescent patterns that kept repeating. In addition, virtually every patient showed fibrinogen (a scablike material) in her lamina propria (that smooth muscle in the interstitium). This was the first definitive hallmark of interstitial cystitis.

At first, we thought these results could have been caused by bacterial infections. Maybe bacteria were causing the antigen-antibody reaction. But urine cultures done at the same time as the biopsy all turned up negative. Cultures for the bacterial venereal disease chlamydia were also negative. Moreover, none of the patients at biopsy was taking suppressive antibiotic therapy; therefore the response was not likely to be a direct result of the antibiotics.

But something had activated the patients' immune systems. What was it? In an attempt to explain these observations, we returned to the patients' charts. And there we found some definite correlations. For example, the tissue of women who had taken only tetracycline therapy turned up with one pattern. Those women who had taken only nitrofurantoin showed another pattern. Women who had taken both antibiotics for a long period showed still another. A much smaller, rare group of women that had not necessarily taken many antibiotics at all showed a different antibody. Another group showed only fibrinogen in the interstitium.

But the question of what a truly normal bladder looks like remained. Virtually all bladder biopsies are taken from people who come to the doctor because something seems to be wrong. Thus no "normal normals" were available for comparison with the findings in my interstitial cystitis patients. I needed to make sure that the immune system is not activated in a healthy bladder by the biopsy technique alone.

I quickly cast my eye toward the operating room nurses at Century City Hospital, where I perform surgery. These nurses were familiar with interstitial cystitis patients. At first they believed, as they had been taught, that this disease was psychosomatic. But as time went on, their attitude changed. Each of them peered through my cystoscope to see the bladder interiors directly. They saw the inflammation, the hemorrhages, the capillary growth, and the ulcerations. And they saw the incredible pain experienced by patients after their bladders had been distended as part of an operative procedure.

And so they volunteered to undergo cystoscopy and bladder biopsies in my office—without anesthesia. The actions of these truly generous and dedicated nurses indicated an enormous trust in me and empathy for the patients. As one of my patients said, "I cry every time I think these nurses did this."

The tissue samples taken from six nurses have served as the normal controls for my continuing studies. There was no fibrinogen in the interstitium of their bladders. Nor did they show signs of antigen-antibody activity.

In addition, we used their tissue to develop a brand-new staining technique that shows what normal and abnormal bladder tissue looks like. Normal tissue has a well-defined thin top layer which represents the GAG secretions that are believed to exist in the bladder (see photographs on p. 88). It came out pink in the staining technique. Underneath was a blue layer (consistent with urothelial cells). Next was a reddish layer (consistent with the interstitium that contained normal amounts of capillaries). The result resembles the NBC peacock.

Abnormal tissue obtained from patients with interstitial cystitis

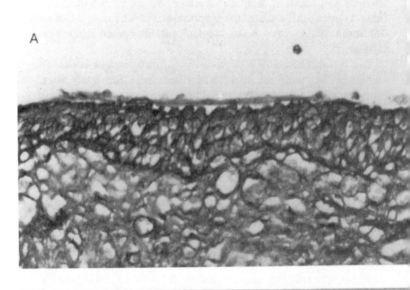

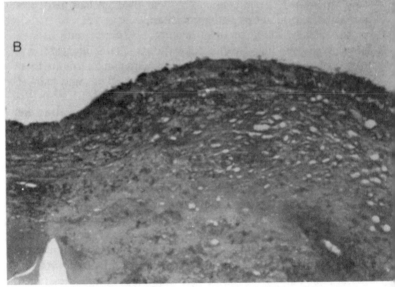

Figure 2-3, (A) Normal bladder. (B) Bladder with interstitial cystitis.

lacked the pink layer. This meant the GAG layer was gone. The blue layer was replaced by a brown material which represented an antibody. And the reddish area of the interstitium was infiltrated by a brown substance (fibrinogen) with huge, dilated, and ruptured capillaries. This staining technique helped to confirm the theory that interstitial cystitis is the result of the loss of the protective layer on the bladder surface.

With the results of this color staining technique, we were able to see that interstitial cystitis is not one disease but many.

Patients with the disease can now be broken down into three major categories. One group of patients has inflammation primarily on the surface of their bladder cells. A second group shows capillary growth and major involvement of their immune systems. A third, those who had fibrinogen only, has cell-mediated disease such as thyroid imbalance.

These results led to the first real diagnostic technique for the diseases that cause interstitial problems. They also led me to think about a new and different concept of autoimmune diseases. The findings indicated that the bladder could be damaged in numerous ways, but they all resulted in a common process called interstitial cystitis, in which the immune system was definitely involved.

Concept: The Role Your Immune System Plays in Interstitial Cystitis

Why should the immune system become chronically activated in a disease such as interstitial cystitis? Granted, a bacterial invasion of the bladder could mount a brief antigen-antibody response, and once the infection was over, the reaction would disappear. However, interstitial cystitis patients do not have bacteria in their bladders.

Physicians have been taught that an autoimmune disease is one in which the immune system turns on itself. Instead of protecting the "self," the body recognizes something of itself as "foreign." Antibodies attack the tissue. Such diseases include arthritis, asthma, and lupus.

This has never made much sense to me. Why would the body destroy itself? I turned the question around: Maybe the body is trying to *protect* itself. Perhaps the immune system, in these diseases, has not gone haywire but rather is attempting some "logical" or adaptive repair.

In interstitial cystitis, the GAG layer is missing or damaged. Urine constantly burns tissue. Nerves are exposed to urine and fire randomly. Capillaries grow continuously. The bladder cramps as it tries to expel urine.

In this theory, the immune system is trying to substitute for the missing GAG layer. It is there to protect or adapt for the tissue's deficient components by placing fibrinogen as the next best impermeable barrier. Fibrinogen serves as the "scab" trying to keep the environment from getting into damaged tissues.

By extension, other autoimmune diseases might be viewed as immunologic adaptations of the body whenever GAG-like layers are damaged. There is a GAG layer in your joints and in your bowels. Could this be implicated in arthritis and colitis? Much more research will have to be done to explore this possibility. The bladder is an excellent organ in which to carry out research because, with instruments, it is readily accessible.

Symptom: Chronic Fatigue

At this point, I was pleased that so many pieces of the puzzle were falling into place. But some patients still didn't fit any of the categories. Many had never taken antibiotics for cystitis, although they may have taken them for acne or other conditions. In any case, antibiotics taken in the absence of infection could not have been a cause in Hunner's day; the drugs hadn't been invented yet. There had to be other factors in the disease that we just had not unearthed.

Margaret had been my patient for a year. One day, she came to tell me that, at long last, she had been diagnosed as having chronic Epstein-Barr virus (EBV) infection. This is the virus that causes mononucleosis. It is very prevalent in our society and 90 percent of the U.S. population has antibodies to it.

But some people such as Margaret, for an unknown reason, have a chronic infection of the virus. The virus remains active in their bodies. Various agents in the environment seem to activate the virus and make it flare up in these unfortunate people, who are predominantly women.

"I'm exhausted all the time," Margaret said. "I have sore

throats, headaches, swollen lymph glands, and a low-grade fever. I know that the virus is the cause of my interstitial cystitis. I know it."

I shook my head no. "That's not possible, Margaret. I've never heard anything about Epstein-Barr virus except that it causes mono. You're telling me that it's not ordinary mono and that you're tired and weak from it?"

But what she said piqued my interest. Other patients had been describing symptoms that sounded like a viral infection. They had headaches, sore throats, and diarrhea. Yet plenty of research had been done trying to relate viruses to interstitial cystitis. All the results had been negative.

Except no one had ever looked at EBV.

"Okay, Margaret," I said. "Just to humor you, I'll test the next five people who walk through my office door for chronic EBV. You'll see. They won't have it."

But they did. They had massive infections.

Concept: Environmental Factors May Trigger Episodes

Very little is known about chronic EBV infections. The virus seems to lie quiescent in the lymph system or in damaged epithelium until something in the environment triggers it to multiply. An infection ensues. Such patients have chronic sore throats and are often given antibiotics for strep throats. Yet their throat tissue is rarely cultured to see if streptococcal bacteria are present.

I theorized that the virus could be responsible for initiating the changes in bladder tissues of interstitial cystitis patients. Such patients would feel fine for a while and then, boom! something would activate the virus and promote the disease we call interstitial cystitis.

Working with EBV authority Dr. Jim Jones, of the National Jewish Center for Immunology & Respiratory Medicine, we came upon one possible agent—phorbol esters. This chemical is used in paints, lacquers, solvents, and a wide range of other industrial chemicals.

More of my patients' symptoms began to make sense. Janie got sick every weekday evening after her husband came home but was fine when he was there on the weekends. The possible reason? He is an automobile mechanic and uses chemicals containing phorbol esters that cling to his clothes. He would bring the chemical into the house after work and Janie's bladder would hurt. On weekends he was free of the chemicals and Janie felt fine.

June got sick when exposed to household cleaners, particularly chlorine bleaches used to whiten sinks. After she hired a cleaning lady, her symptoms improved.

Nancy noticed her bladder hurt every time she went to the manicurist. Phorbol esters are in the glues and polishes used by beauticians to create that long-nail look. Nancy stopped having her nails done.

Probably there are many environmental factors that precipitate EBV to reactivate and multiply, causing the chronic symptoms of some interstitial cystitis patients. The whole question is being researched under the auspices of the Interstitial Cystitis Foundation.

Symptom: Menstruation, Menopause, Pregnancy Coinciding with Flare-ups

Cathy's bladder began to hurt five days before her period and it kept hurting until twenty-four hours after she started to menstruate. It happened every month. "It's a dull aching toward the base of my bladder," she said.

Estelle's interstitial cystitis had responded well to treatment. She could travel again and her life was back to normal. Then, as she entered menopause, her gynecologist gave her a combination estrogen and progesterone therapy. Her bladder pain returned with a vengeance.

Marlene had had bladder problems since she was eighteen. When she was twenty-five, she got pregnant, and to her astonishment, her symptoms disappeared. She had a blissful pregnancy. Then, six weeks after the delivery, the bladder pain came back worse than it had ever been.

Concept: How Cycles Alter Bladder Behavior

Perhaps in this complicated disease, equally complicated hormonal factors come into play. Women develop interstitial cystitis far more frequently than men—at a ratio of 100 to 1. Men do not have monthly hormonal cycles. Maybe there are clues to be found in this fact.

It has been shown that estrogen increases the GAG layer and presumed that progesterone decreases it. Thus women would be susceptible to membrane leak and bladder pain when progesterone levels are high. This maximum occurs twenty-four hours before the onset of menstruation.

It fits Cathy's symptoms to a T. For two weeks before her period, as her progesterone levels rose, she gradually developed urinary frequency. Her urinary pH rose to 7.5, indicating leaking cellular membranes. When her period came, she felt relief. Her pH fell back to normal range and she felt fine until the next time she ovulated.

Estelle was fine until she took progesterone at menopause. It may have destabilized her bladder and caused her symptoms of frequency to recur.

Marlene's entire hormonal balance changed during pregnancy. Six weeks after she delivered, however, her bladder problems resumed. The protective effects of estrogen were gone.

It may be that some women have naturally immature GAG layers. This would predispose them, from birth, to factors that alter bladder GAGs. I call them members of the teeny-weeny bladder club.

The complex effects of hormones and subhormones on bladder tissue during menstrual cycles is an area that needs much more investigation. It is another area of research by the Interstitial Cystitis Foundation.

An Environmental Disease

In six years of work on interstitial cystitis, my patients and I have uncovered many factors contributing to painful bladder syndrome. We've seen how antibiotics taken in the absence of infection, hormonal cycles, Epstein-Barr virus, scarlet fever, and foods or drugs that increase serotonin production can affect the GAG layer.

But the mystery is not solved. The puzzle has many missing pieces. Why, for example, do cases of interstitial cystitis cluster in an Indiana neighborhood? Women from the same block have the disease while women across town do not.

Why does a woman who moved next door to a landfill in New Jersey suddenly develop bladder pain and why do kids on her block suffer nosebleeds? What have they been exposed to?

Doctors working in California's Central Valley have reported clusters of interstitial cystitis patients in areas known for pesticide contamination of ground water. Is there a link? Maybe. Maybe not.

Radon is an invisible gas that is released from rock containing radioactive elements. Such rocks are abundant in many parts of the United States and have been used in building the foundations of numerous homes. Epidemiologists have recently shown that exposure to radon gas correlates with lung cancer. We may find a similar but different agent that relates to interstitial cystitis.

Literally hundreds of agents could be implicated in the prevalence of interstitial cystitis around the world. One would expect the incidence to vary from country to country, as it does, since different environmental factors are at play.

The work I do never seems to stop. There is an ever evolving understanding of cell membranes and how to stabilize them. No single method will make everyone well. We are engaged in a great mystery hunt. Each patient must observe her symptoms and environment to see what triggers or ameliorates an attack. That way, we can keep filling in missing pieces of the interstitial cystitis puzzle.

THREE

Interstitial Cystitis: Clues for Getting a Correct Diagnosis and Treatment Plan

If you were to come to me for a diagnosis of interstitial cystitis, we would look for numerous indications. In my opinion, the symptoms known as urethritis can be an early sign of the disease. To have interstitial cystitis, you do not have to have a shrunken, ulcerated bladder. I maintain that if lost bladder capacity were the only hallmark of interstitial cystitis, 77 percent of my patients with the disease would never be diagnosed as having it. If I depended on just one factor in making a diagnosis, I would miss many patients. For example, Marilyn went to a leading urologist for help with her symptoms of constant bladder burn. He refused to treat her, however, because she did not have urinary pain. He said flatly that she did not have interstitial cystitis.

The first step to diagnosis, of course, is to take your medical history.

- What diseases have you had?
- What problems, if any, run in your family?
- When did your symptoms begin?
- Have you noticed what agents make you feel better or worse?
- Do you have digestive problems?
- Are you a chronic dieter?

Next we would take a urine sample and run some tests. We would want to make sure you do not have an infection. We would note your urine pH. If it is alkaline, I would like to know if you take calcium supplements that are buffered with bicarbonate. If you do not, a highly alkaline urine could be a sign of interstitial cystitis.

We would draw blood and measure your white blood cell count. A low count would indicate that your immune system has been activated. We would test for Epstein-Barr virus activity, and thyroid function.

Once all this information is collected, I usually can tell within 98 percent certainty whether or not you will have interstitial cystitis. But to determine which type, I must look directly into your bladder and obtain tissue for the various tests we've described.

This has to be done in the hospital operating room. For people with healthy bladders, a cystoscopic procedure can be done in the office. But for those with interstitial cystitis, cystoscopy is unthinkable without general anesthesia. The pain of distending the bladder could not be tolerated by a conscious patient.

The cystoscope is a lighted tubular instrument that I insert into your bladder. I would first look for visual signs of angiogenesis, those corkscrewlike capillaries. After filling the bladder to full capacity with water, I would drain it and measure the volume. This tells me your true capacity and from it we can calculate your normal voiding range. Generally healthy people void at about half of their anatomic capacity.

I would look to see if the last bit of water draining from your bladder contains any blood. More importantly, when I look back in, are there bleeding sites, hemorrhages, striations (streaks), or even ulcerations on your tissue?

The next step is to photograph your bladder. I do this for every patient. It gives us a record of what your bladder looked like when you were first diagnosed.

I would then snip out some tissue for immunofluorescence and the staining technique described in Chapter Two. This will help us determine which variety of interstitial cystitis you have and help tailor therapy.

At this point, I would also start you on a basic treatment I have devised to help your bladder tissue heal in the face of a hostile environment—that is, your urine.

Regenerating Bladder Cells

In thinking about leaky cell membranes (see Figure 2-1, Leaky Urothelial Cell, p. 71), I began by looking for ways to stabilize cells. How might one stop the membrane from interacting with urine?

It has been demonstrated that cells duplicate, divide, and grow when the intracellular pH (that is, the pH within the cell) increases to above 7.2. Classic studies of sea urchin eggs show this dramatically. When the eggs are placed in a medium with a high pH, they duplicate and begin regeneration all by themselves, without fertilization.

My approach to interstitial cystitis was inspired by this natural phenomenon. I reasoned that the bladder cells of interstitial cystitis patients had been burned by acid. Therefore the intracellular pH was no longer in the correct range. If I could raise the pH above 7.2, the damaged cells could at least have a fighting chance to regenerate. They might begin to repair themselves naturally because pH-dependent enzymes and other metabolic intermediates in the cell could then begin functioning. This is akin to throwing on the switch to the generator inside a bladder cell. But how to turn on the cells, how to raise their pH when the tissue is still exposed to the very environment that is destroying it?

Since 1978, a by-product of the paper industry has been approved for the treatment of interstitial cystitis. The drug is called *dimethyl sulfoxide,* or DMSO. Although it was not a cure for the disease, it was found to offer symptomatic relief for many patients. As time wore on, however, the beneficial effects of DMSO would lessen. Often the drug seemed just to stop working.

I began to investigate other properties of DMSO. Researchers had found that DMSO can penetrate normal barriers, even skin, and quickly get into tissue. And if DMSO were combined with other drugs, the DMSO would piggyback those drugs directly into tissue. As such, DMSO was a natural transport mechanism for carrying drugs into the body. One group of researchers, for example, found that a steroid drug mixed with DMSO could be transported into tissue at one one-thousandth the dosage required systemically.

Moreover, DMSO itself only exerted transient effects on tissues it penetrated. In all of the diseases for which it was tried there were no long-lasting effects. But if you consider it to be a carrier, not a treatment in itself, DMSO could be very handy.

My goal was to stop inflammation and raise intracellular pH in your damaged bladder cells. The first criterion could be met with steroids, anti-inflammatory drugs used widely to help stabilize membranes of the body. But DMSO and steroids alone will not do the trick. Steroids require an alkaline pH to remain active. When placed in the bladder, acid in urine can easily inactivate a steroid, resulting in no prolonged effect on bladder tissue. Therefore a buffer was required. The obvious answer lay in a box of Arm & Hammer baking soda.

Bicarbonate of soda, as noted, is alkaline and helps stabilize the tissue of burn patients. Also, sea urchins require bicarbonate to raise pH so they can multiply and divide. By incorporating sodium bicarbonate into the mixture, I could hope to buffer the steroid and induce cellular regeneration.

Thus the Gillespie cocktail was born. Placing this trio of drugs—DMSO, steroid, and sodium bicarbonate—into the bladders of interstitial cystitis patients had dramatic results. In one subset of patients, those who were only missing the protective GAG layer, the bladder tissue stabilized within a few weeks.

This treatment has also proved effective for patients with what is called radiation cystitis. Molly, for example, was cured of cancer of the cervix through intense radiation therapy. The treatment stopped one disease and started another—namely, interstitial cystitis. Molly's bladder lining was severely damaged by the radiation. She experienced pain, burning, cramping, frequency, and other hallmarks of interstitial cystitis. She saw many doctors before I made the diagnosis of radiation cystitis because Molly simply neglected to tell her doctors that she had been treated for cervical cancer with radiation. I found out from the questionnaire she filled out and treated her, successfully, with the Gillespie cocktail.

How Can We Arrest Abnormal Capillary Growth?

There were patients, however, whose bladder tissue was more severely damaged. Although helped by this cocktail, they did not remain stabilized. These were women who showed massive capillary growth, or angiogenesis, in the bladder. They tested positive for one particular antibody within these very same capillaries.

The capillaries of the interstitium serve as a filtration mechanism for the contents of urine and extracellular fluid; they drain away impurities. In one subset of interstitial cystitis patients, this filtering mechanism is out of balance. They experienced continuous capillary proliferation.

A different treatment approach was therefore needed to stabilize them. This led to an investigational protocol that I developed with the Food and Drug Administration, to use a new drug called Angiostat. Pamela Sue Martin was the first person to receive this unique medication.

"Ever since my treatments, I've been fine," Pamela said recently. "Only when I'm under severe stress do I feel little twinges, but nothing like it used to be. But now I understand what is going on in my body. I stay on a low-acid diet. I know how to reduce stress. And I can keep myself healthy."

How the Environment Can Aggravate Your Immune System

When Teddy Epstein discovered the Epstein-Barr virus in the 1950s, he said he felt it would be the Rosetta stone of cancer. I believe it may be the code breaker of inflammatory disease as well.

EBV is the most common cause of infectious mononucleosis. It makes you tired and weak and your lymph nodes swell. After two months, your immune system inactivates the virus. You develop antibodies that prevent reinfection.

Or so it is with most people. Some people have chronic, constant infections. The diagnosis can be made by looking at what are called blood titres, which are measures of infection in blood.

EBV Titres

There are four aspects of EBV titres:

• The IgG titre tells us whether or not you have ever been exposed to the virus. If positive, you probably had mono at one time and recovered. You are supposedly immune to it.

• The IgM titre indicates recent infection. You most probably had this infection within the past six weeks.

• The early capsid antigen titre tells us you have active disease at the moment. The virus is busy duplicating in your body.

• Finally, the Epstein-Barr nuclear antigen (ebna) titre tells us your disease is at least several months old.

If you were to test 1,000 people at random, 90 percent would show IgG and ebna titres. But, as we have recently discovered, many interstitial cystitis patients show chronic active titres. That is, they have titres showing previous exposure (IgG and ebna) plus early capsid antigen titres. The virus has become reactivated.

How the virus gets reactivated is a current area of medical research. We know this virus can live in damaged epithelium, the special protective cells that line cavities and organs such as the lungs and bladder. What fascinates me is that interstitial cystitis patients have a large epithelial organ, the bladder, which is damaged.

What does the virus do to interstitial cystitis patients? Let's assume the virus is in your bladder tissue. It rests there quietly, without mishap, until something comes along to activate it. Such activators may be substances, such as phorbol esters and other chemicals, from the environment. The substance stimulates the virus to go from a quiescent to an active, destructive phase. In the quiescent phase the virus "sits back." In the destructive phase, it ruptures cells and destroys them.

One patient got sick within fifteen minutes after arriving at work every day. She then discovered that her office shared an air conditioning duct with two neighboring cabinetry shops. The chemicals they used on furniture wafted into her office and activated her virus. Blood tests revealed high early capsid antigen titres. When she went home at night she soon felt better.

But the toll on her was emotionally devastating. She grew more and more depressed, more and more tired. Like so many interstitial cystitis patients, she thought her life was out of control. She even thought of suicide.

Therapies That Hurt More than Help

Because patients are so often desperate, urologists have tried some fairly drastic therapies to treat interstitial cystitis, therapies that in my opinion tend to do more harm than good. For example, although I am trained and certified to use lasers in the treatment of bladder disease, I have found this technique to have no lasting benefit. A laser is basically a fancy instrument used to cauterize tissue. Ulcerated portions of the bladder are simply "burned" away. But this process actually creates more damage to bladder tissue and increases capillary growth. Lasers are not a satisfactory way to deal with interstitial cystitis.

Another therapy is called bladder augmentation. Basically, the top of the bladder is lopped off surgically. Only the bladder neck, trigone, and ureters are left. Then a piece of bowel is excised and refashioned to form a new top half of the bladder. The goal is to restore bladder capacity in patients whose bladders are shrunken and scarred from years of unarrested interstitial cystitis.

Bladder augmentations do work for a small percentage of patients, namely those who do not have disease in the base of their natural bladders. But for most patients, this is not the case. They get the "new" bladder, only to find that their "old" symptoms of burning, frequency, and pain have not been alleviated. They then wind up with two different membrane surfaces in their bladders. It becomes very difficult to apply cell stabilization techniques to this hybrid tissue. The outlook for many "augmented" patients is not good.

The last resort for some women is total cystectomy, or removal of the bladder itself. The ureters are joined and made to drain passively through a hole on the stomach. Urine is collected in a bag that is drained periodically.

When a woman with interstitial cystitis comes to me for treatment, I make her a promise: I will never, under any circumstances, remove her bladder. (It may well be, however, that her disease is so far progressed or her bladder has been so damaged that I cannot stop the disease process and cannot save her bladder. In these rare instances, cystectomy may be the only answer.) The reason I make this promise to patients is that I am bound and determined to find a way to stabilize every bladder that crosses my doorstep. A patient needs to know this, so we can work together to solve her particular piece of the mystery of what causes interstitial cystitis.

My orientation to this disease is to discover the cellular nature of it. I try to arrest the process and give you back control over your life.

What the Mind Can Do to Help Heal the Body

Whatever the cause of your interstitial cystitis, you are faced with the daily task of coping with this devastating disease. It is not easy.

A few of my patients, in fact, are clinical psychologists. But even though they are experts in helping people resolve problems, they were unable to apply their training to help themselves.

Martha, for example, refused to look me in the face on her first three visits. How she dealt with her own patients at this time still mystifies me. As a practicing psychologist, she had convinced herself that her pain was psychosomatic. She underwent sex therapy to try to cope with the pain of intercourse. She worked every minute of the day to dissociate her body from her mind.

After several treatments, however, she changed. She looked me in the face. She smiled. And she admitted that the pain had driven her to avoid facing the world about her, including her patients, her family, and her physician.

I have watched many patients undergo such changes, transforming from destitute, emotional cripples into functioning adult women.

My goal is to give each patient back the control over her life. I ask her to be responsible for her own health. It requires a lot of work on her part. In talking to patients about coping with interstitial cystitis, I am reminded of a story my mother told me when I was a schoolgirl:

Once there were two frogs that had fallen into a pail of cream. The sides were slippery and steep so that despite all their efforts, they could not escape the pail. One frog decided it was hopeless. She gave up, sank to the bottom, and drowned. The second frog refused to give up. She kept churning away with all her strength. Suddenly, she let out a satisfied croak because there she was, sitting on a pat of butter churned up through her own efforts.

If you believe, as some interstitial cystitis patients do, that there is no hope for a cure, you will sink to the bottom and psychologically drown in your own sorrow. But if you take each day and decide that you're not going to let the disease conquer you, you will find a way to get on top of your own pat of butter.

Anger won't help. Some interstitial cystitis patients are furious with the medical profession for not having solved the puzzle of this disease. I believe anger is a self-defeating emotion. You cannot change your disease by ranting at people who treated you, in good faith, years ago. Medical knowledge changes over time. So I encourage you to put your anger behind you and concentrate on today.

Will There Ever Be a Cure?

I had a patient with interstitial cystitis who came into the office recently and the first thing she said was, "Is there a cure for this? What is the cure?" I had to sit her down and give her my "Semantics of Cure" lecture.

"What does the word *cure* really mean?" I asked her.

She said, "Well, it means your problem is gone forever."

"Does it mean there is no evidence that the problem ever existed?" I wondered.

"Oh," she said. "When you put it that way, there is no cure for anything."

"Exactly right. There is no cure that eradicates all evidence that a disease was ever there. The cure for appendicitis is an appendectomy, but you still have the scar. For every medical problem, the best a physician can do is to help you gain control over it."

I do not like the word *cure*. My goal is to have you, the patient, control the disease process rather than having the disease process control you. Your goal is to resume a normal life. To do so, you must take responsibility for your health. But if you consider yourself "cured," you might well go out and undo all the things that made your bladder stable. You might think, "I'm completely well. I can eat what I like, take diet pills, use any antibiotic because I'm cured!" And, of course, by exposing your bladder to harmful environmental factors you could start the disease process all over again.

The patient who came into my office asking for a cure failed to understand that the power to heal was in herself. Thus, she set herself up as the Victim.

How to Stop Being a "Victim"

Throughout this book, I have not used the word *victim*. I do not buy into the idea that women with interstitial cystitis have been victimized by the medical profession or by life in general. The women who come to me with the need to be treated as victims are the ones I cannot help; I will never be able to help them until they learn to break the trap of self-victimization and take responsibility for their own health.

On the other hand, I can understand why they feel this way. People with chronic pain, especially when it lasts over six months, sometimes tap into very primal needs. But the victim mentality is self-defeating. The victim has capitulated to the disease. She may even begin to rely on her role as victim for a sense of self-worth.

I urge you to examine your feelings about interstitial cystitis, should you have this disease. Victimization encourages anger, which will get you nowhere. Victimization encourages self-pity and lack of responsibility. When you view yourself as a victim, you are doing nothing to help yourself.

And there are, as you have seen in this and the previous chapter, many things you can do to begin to help yourself. While there is no "cure" for interstitial cystitis, there are dozens of ways you can help yourself, medically and psychologically.

Virginia

Virginia has run several group therapy sessions of interstitial cystitis patients in the Los Angeles area. As a marriage and family psychotherapist with the disease, she understands interstitial cystitis in a way that most urologists do not. I think you should read her story:

"I had a lot of pain the first year. But unfortunately for me, I had a mother who was a hypochondriac. She loved every illness. And I was so determined that I would not also become a hypochondriac that I assumed the pain was all in my mind: I must be crazy; they could not find anything wrong with me.

"So I started a search. I would figure out why my psyche was harming my soma. I would be the clever psychologist and cure myself. Whenever I came to the end of a day, completely exhausted, I would say, 'Yes, it's true, I'm not dealing well with life.'

"The search continued through years of therapy until I finally began to realize, 'Wait a minute. I am not a crazy human being. I hurt. There is pain.'

"So I started a new search. I went to physician after physician. My husband was absolutely convinced that I was a hypochondriac like my mother. Our relationship began to develop a lot of problems.

"Even though I was a therapist and I felt psychologically okay, I began to have suicidal thoughts. I began to think I could only go through so many more bad weeks, then if I cannot find relief, I want to die. For me, the important thing is not the length of life we live; it is the quality of life. And I want quality. I want to dance. I want to play and have fun.

"One day my husband saw Dr. Gillespie on television and he called me. 'C'mere. This is what you have. Listen to what she's saying.'

"I listened hard and the next day went to my urologist and explained to him what I had heard. And he said, 'Oh, that's a horrible disease. You don't want it.'

"Now, he's a lovely man. He said, 'Okay, I'll put some DMSO into you. If it helps that will be fine. We'll go from there.' He put in some DMSO and it really helped. But when it came time to go back, I decided to try Dr. Gillespie herself.

"After we went through the full diagnosis and she told me what it was, I cried. I started sobbing because of the years and years I had thought I was nuts, headed for the loony bin, knowing no one could find anything. I think I cried for a week.

"But next there was a feeling of absolute relief that someone had heard my agony. Someone had heard my pain. I was not nuts. And there was hope.

"Then the fear started. The anguish, not out of sadness, but out of the knowledge I have something really unknown. My first response was, 'Well, the understanding of this disease is in its infancy stage. We don't know what we're going to do. I'll probably be a guinea pig.

"But then I did what psychologists do. I reframed the issue. I thought, 'Isn't this wonderful! My disease was found out when research is just beginning so I can be in on the adventure. I'm going to get well!'

"But then I locked into a new psychological trap. In getting my first treatments of the Gillespie cocktail, I locked on to the phrase 'six weeks.' Instead of hearing Dr. Gillespie say, 'The first course is six weeks,' I heard instead, 'It will be cured in six weeks.' I wanted it to be over in six weeks. And of course, it was not over so quickly. But it was much better.

"The next lesson I learned was how to deal with setbacks. This happened to me when I experienced a potassium loss and had to stop treatments until my potassium levels could be restored to normal.

"I felt real terror. 'Oh, my God, I may never get back into control.' All the questions about how to deal with this disease came back. And then I had another setback, an infection. Every time I had a setback, I tried to fight the feelings I was having. I tried to say, 'I'm not depressed! I'm going to lick this.'

"Then I tried a new tactic. I had read literature suggesting that people who handle disease with a sense of anger or a sense of positive well-being do better than others. Accordingly, I decided to deal with my depression. I was furious. I was wallowing in depression. And I called it a snit day. I am allowed to have snits. For twenty-four hours that I'm depressed, I allow myself to feel sad. I don't try to tell people I'm okay when I'm not. If my husband doesn't like it that day, I suggest he go into another room. Because if I'm going to be in a snit, I'm going to be in a snit. When I finally realized that depression is only anger directed at yourself, it only took twenty-four hours to return to normal.

"And I began to understand that even in my snits, I was better off than in the earlier days of my disease. I had whole nights when I could sleep. I had days without pain. Was that not glorious?"

Interstitial cystitis patients like Virginia have done remarkably well. They are also willing to extend a hand to others, to help them cope with the stress of this disease. But in so doing, many have noticed an odd psychological problem. When women who are not doing well talk to women who are doing well with this disease, communication can break down. It is as if some patients do not want to hear that others are doing well. They feel anger, jealousy, and fear. Why is she better and not me?

On the other hand, my patients say some women they talk to (who were not diagnosed, treated, and educated at my clinic) seem not to be willing to take responsibility for their own health. "A woman called me from Boston," said Judy, "wanting to know how I was doing. I told her about all the things I have done and she didn't want to listen. She wanted to complain."

On the other hand, some interstitial cystitis patients who are stabilized want to forget this whole miserable episode of life. They refuse to talk to women who are not doing well because it reminds them of their former agony.

I believe we should all support one another. Those who do well should help those in pain. The women in pain should not resent those who do well.

The Leaping Frog Society

There is always hope and there are people who have been freed from the ravages of interstitial cystitis. In fact, my patients who remain free of symptoms for six months or longer have formed the Leaping Frog Society. At this writing, six of them have become pregnant and delivered healthy babies. Several others have sent in their wedding announcements. They all churned up their pat of butter and got out of that slippery pail. As their stories reveal, it was not an easy journey.

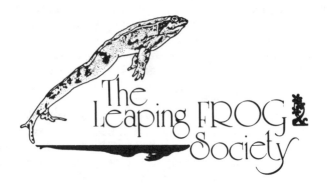

The Leaping FROG Society

Paula

About six years ago I started to have burning in my bladder. I thought it was an infection and trotted off to the urologist. He said it was typical for women my age to have a little pain in the bladder caused by stress. He then gave me thirteen silver nitrate treatments. Even though these hurt a great deal, he kept giving them to me. And I got worse.

For the next two or three years, I felt so much pressure and burning that I lived on pain pills. Many days I could not get out of bed. I saw three more urologists. The fourth one told me my pain was all in my head. He said I was basically crazy and would have to accept that.

Finally, as I was too sick to get out of bed for months, my gynecologist said I needed a hysterectomy. He thought I might have endometriosis. But before surgery, he sent me to a famous urologist for a workup. This, the fifth urologist, performed cystoscopy under anesthesia. Later, he told me, "The good news is that you do not have cancer, you have a normal bladder." My gynecologist had mentioned the term interstitial cystitis and I asked the urologist about it. He said it was such a rare disease that I could not possibly have it.

So at age thirty-nine I had a hysterectomy. Everything came out. I felt better for three months and then the pain came back. I was devastated. I went back to the urologist and had a second cystoscopy. He looked me in the eye and said, "There is nothing I can do for you."

About this time my internist gave me antidepressants and I went back to bed, unable to walk because of the pain. Then I saw an article about interstitial cystitis and Dr. Gillespie's clinic. I took the article to my internist with tears in my eyes. He said, "You are one of those women who will keep going from doctor to doctor, looking for an answer you will never find." He, too, thought it was all in my head.

I began treatment with Dr. Gillespie and slowly improved. It was not an overnight miracle. We tried different things and had to keep working on it. I'd say it took eighteen months for my symptoms to be brought under control.

And I can say today that I am pain-free. I am beginning to eat some of the foods that I could not eat before. It's such an unbelievable feeling that I think I should knock on wood so as not to break my good fortune. But I know, deep inside, it was not luck that made me better. It was hard work.

Esther

I developed a burning in my bladder in August 1981. It did not feel like the cystitis I had had before so I went to a urologist. He dilated my urethra which did not help at all. It made me worse.

The second urologist told me my symptoms could be connected with incipient multiple sclerosis. He gave me antibiotics and Valium. Neither helped.

The third urologist insinuated I had sexual problems with my husband and that this was the cause of my bladder pain. I have been happily married for twenty-five years and couldn't believe he was saying such a thing. He sent me to a biofeedback therapist and began treatments with DMSO and silver nitrate. None of it helped.

I flew to other cities and saw top specialists in my search for help. One, a leader among all urologists, told me that it sounded like interstitial cystitis but that without the symptom of frequency (I only had burning) I could not possibly have interstitial cystitis.

I have always loved to entertain. But for over two years I could not do anything. I resigned from all my volunteer work and spent the days lying down with a heating pad. I had a hysterectomy.

And the bladder pain continued. I must say I resented it. It completely interfered with normal life. I could not trust myself to feel well and was afraid to plan anything. If I had a dinner party, I might have to leave in the middle of it and go lie down. And the way the doctors treated me was humiliating.

When I first went to Dr. Gillespie, I was contrite. I had always been told I was creating this illness. I told her I felt helpless, humiliated, and that maybe I was losing my mind. And she said, "The problem is not in your head. You're sitting on it." I couldn't believe her at first. I had been to the so-called top specialists in the country. And she then proceeded to prove it to me.

I am definitely improved. I can entertain and go on family ski trips. I'm not yet cured in the sense that there is never any discomfort. But the quality of my life has returned. The feeling is wonderful.

Amelia

I had interstitial cystitis for twelve years. Over much of that time I was treated at an excellent, nearby diagnostic clinic—excellent, that is, for most diseases except interstitial cystitis. In all the time I went there, they never explained my disease to me. They always said the same thing: "You are doing well. Keep up the good work." They suggested hydraulic stretching of my bladder to make it bigger.

Meanwhile, I had reached a point of desperation. I asked my doctors if there was something more we could do. All the medications I had taken were not making my bladder well. I took opium suppositories for pain near the rectum. It was so bad that I could not sit or stand any pressure in that area.

Also, the disease was so erratic. There were days when it got better and days when it was excruciating. I asked what about diet? Is it something I am doing? Is it something I'm eating or drinking? They would always assure me it had nothing to do with food. It was then that my doctors described different kinds of surgery. The alternative was to remove my bladder or augment it with bowel. The very thought of surgery put me into a terrible depression.

About this time, a friend saw Pamela Sue Martin on television talking about her bladder problem. I called the station and they

Letters

A LETTER FROM MARY ANN

It's been one year this month since I finished the treatments for interstitial cystitis and I can't tell you how wonderful it's been to have a pain-free bladder. I didn't write any sooner because I wanted to make sure that tomorrow wouldn't be different. This is the first pain-free year I've had in at least ten or fifteen years.

A LETTER FROM MOLLY

I have felt better in the last five months since coming to your clinic July 10th than I have in about seventeen years. Now I believe in miracles. I tell my friends and family I am like a song, "I Have a New Body, Praise the Lord, I Have a New Life." As I told you, a famous urologist in Texas had told me I had to have my bladder removed. A neighbor's son talked to four urologists for me and they said that it was all I could do for an advanced case like mine. Now, after your treatments, I have gone from about 1/3 cup capacity to 3/4 cup capacity.

A LETTER FROM CEILA

I think we each must have within us the power of curing. It takes strong faith. The doctors are there to help us.

A LETTER FROM ALMA

This was the best Christmas I had in a long time. I actually enjoyed the rush of shopping!

gave me Dr. Gillespie's name and address. I called and talked to her nurse, who explained the basic treatments to me and the attention I would have to pay to diet and vitamins.

Since I live in New England and Dr. Gillespie was so far away, my husband suggested I simply get some DMSO treatments from a local physician. But I was fascinated by the diet connection. I wanted to go to California and get the whole story for myself. In October 1984 I made my first visit to her clinic.

As I was waking up from the anesthesia after my first treatment with the Gillespie cocktail I remember feeling horribly groggy. I asked, "Is my bladder worth saving?" She said, "You bet it is!" and I felt incredible relief. The talk of surgery had really frightened me. She assured me that I could keep my bladder and she helped set things up with another urologist near me who would continue treatments under her guidance. My hometown urologist said the treatments made a lot of sense. He was happy to do them.

In the meantime I started to watch my diet. I saw there was a definite relationship between pain and foods. I love fresh tomatoes in season. It was nothing for me to eat three or four a day out of the garden. I used to drink iced tea with lots of lemon.

Now I have not had anything acidic for over a year. Although I still have the disease, I feel wonderful. Now I know I'm healing.

I did have one setback, however. I developed terrible pain and assumed my interstitial cystitis had come back forever. It turned out I had a real, bacterial infection. Once it cleared up, I was back to a more normal condition. I know I am making progress now.

Denise

I have now had eleven months of treatment on Dr. Gillespie's oral protocol. On a scale of one to ten, with ten feeling the best you ever have in your life, I'd say I'm a seven or eight. This is fantastic. I went back to exercising and taking aerobics four times a week. The constant yeast infections I've always had are now gone. And some really good news is that I now have normal sex without fear of being hurt.

FOUR

How to Talk
So Your Doctor
Will Listen

I like to go to the waiting room to greet each patient and escort her personally into my office. In this way, I let the patient know that she is coming to someone who wants to help her in solving her urological problem as a partner.

If you were my patient and it was your first visit, I would put you to work before we talked. When you come in, my nurse would hand you a three-page questionnaire. It is geared to give me basic information, helping me orient and organize my thinking about you as a patient. And it forces you to organize your thoughts and orient yourself as a partner in our consultation.

Although the questionnaire is simple, if you are like some of my patients, it may take you a half hour to fill it out. To me, this indicates you have not prepared yourself enough ahead of time. You should organize your thoughts and make a list. Be prepared.

Believe in Lists

You probably don't go to the grocery store without a shopping list. Why shouldn't the same be true for a doctor's visit?

It seems that many physicians have been taught to beware of patients carrying lists because list makers have a reputation for being phobic. It is not known where this stereotype originated but recently, a family practitioner from Alabama, Dr. John F. Burnum, debunked it in the prestigious *New England Journal of Medicine*. The *Journal* rarely runs nonscientific articles, but Dr. Burnum's article was anecdotal, based on his own observations that list-writing patients were quite sane. The editors believed the subject extremely important and thus ran the article as a way of alerting physicians to this point of view.

"Traditional medical wisdom holds that patients who relate their complaints to their physicians from lists are, ipso facto, emotionally ill," Dr. Burnum wrote. "DeGowin and DeGowin in their venerable textbook on diagnosis say that note writing is 'almost a sure sign of psychoneurosis. The patient with organic disease does not require references to written notes to give the essence of his story.' " But, said Dr. Burnum, "Note writing is a normal, honorable practice that can be used to advantage in patient care."

Dr. Burnum decided to observe seventy-two list-writing patients. "I found no association of emotional disorders with list writing in men," he reported. "Women list writers are more apt to have nervous troubles, but the majority were emotionally normal. Almost all of these emotionally normal list writers had serious physical disorders. Patients with organic disease, therefore, do refer to written notes to give the essence of their story—and not because they are peculiar or crazy."

Note writers simply want to get things straight, he said. Even though they may be anxious and distraught, they are nevertheless seeking clarity, order, information, and control, and to avoid wasting the doctor's time.

Most lists seen by Dr. Burnum consisted of the patient's symptoms and logical questions they wanted to ask. Most contained five or six items, but an emotionally stable executive had written a twenty-point list.

"Lists comprise the same thousand-and-one subjects discussed by all patients: skin blemishes, gas, chest pain, My sister has cancer, do I? shots for foreign travel, Why does my blood pressure fluctuate? family or job troubles, diet, vitamins, medications and exercise," Dr. Burnum said.

"Notes may be of great help in the orderly transfer of information to the physician. Medical care turns on communication. Whatever helps patients express themselves and helps physicians understand patients is acceptable."

I agree wholeheartedly with Dr. Burnum. Many list-writing patients do have complicated disorders. It takes time to diagnose such cases and it requires considerable skill on the part of the physician to interview such patients.

In fact, many physicians do not know how to coax patients into revealing important information—especially small things that the patient may think are inconsequential but which turn out to reveal aspects of a disease process. In medicine, as in other walks of life, there are few skilled interviewers.

I have my own little black binder in which I keep daily lists, projected lists, lists of unfinished work, and lists of concepts and ideas. When a patient bearing a list comes to see me, I take it as a sign of how complicated her disease process has become and how well prepared the patient is.

One extraordinary patient put together a virtual book on her disease, complete with index tabs. It included her medical history, copies of her lab tests, her independent observations, things other doctors had done, her husband's views, lists of questions, and treatments tried.

When she took this compendium to one well-known urologist, he refused to look at it. When she brought it to me, I asked for my own copy so I could underline parts, refer to it, and use it in arriving at a diagnosis. It indeed held the key to her problem, which was treated, and she is now pain-free and doing very well.

You don't have to go to this extent in making lists but coming prepared to every office visit makes economic and medical sense.

How Women Can Get the Best Help: The FEMALE Formula

Here's what you need to get organized when preparing for a visit to the doctor. Remember the "FEMALE" formula. Each letter stands for an important aspect of preparing to establish a successful partnership with your physician:

- *F*acts
- *E*volution
- *M*edications
- *A*ssociated problems
- *L*aboratory records
- *E*motion

Facts

Before you go to the store to spend your money, you sit down and assess what you really need. Before going to a physician, you should assess what you really want the doctor to do for you. What do you need from this physician and how are you going to get it? Do you need an investigator to unravel a mystery, or does the problem seem pretty clear?

You should be organized when you go. As you would take an inventory of what's in your cupboard before shopping, you should take an inventory of what you've observed. Identify the facts by thinking about these questions:

- Tell me, does it hurt before, after, or while you urinate?
- Does it hurt at night or is it associated with lifting, coughing, running, sneezing, or jogging?
- Is there a burning sensation associated with voiding?
- Is there a pressure or cramp?
- Where is the pain located, what causes it, what relieves it?
- Does it get better or worse when you eat certain foods?
- What is the color of your urine?
- Is there debris in your urine?
- Have you seen blood in the urine or is the blood only on the tissue paper when you wipe?
- Do you get pain down your leg? Do you have lower back problems? Do you have pains that go into your hip, your leg, up your spine?
- Do you leak urine when you run or jump in place, cough, or sneeze or does it leak all the time?
- Do you get fevers with any of the symptoms you're describing? Have you recorded those temperatures?
- Do you have a watery green discharge from the vagina as a symptom or is there a thick, cottage cheese–like material?
- Has your sexual partner had any problems?

• Do you get infections whether or not you have intercourse?
• Do you void with a good stream? Does it stop and start?
• Does it burn on the outside of the urethra or in the vagina when you void?
• Does it feel like your insides are falling out?

I know that women are extremely accurate observers of fact. They are very aware, in great detail, of what hurts them. But many of the facts might not get through to the doctor unless you have thought them out and written them down ahead of time.

Evolution

Once you have put down the facts, it is important to note the chronological evolution of your symptoms. This will help us find out how your problems may have come about. I begin interviewing each patient with, "You were perfectly fine until . . . ?" I want her to focus on when her body started to change.

I get many surprising answers. One woman immediately realized, with the help of her husband, that her problem began four years earlier than she had thought. She had thought her problem started after she took medication prescribed by a doctor the year before. Her husband recalled that while they were out camping four years earlier, she had needed to void frequently and was tired for several weeks. Her problem, we eventually found, was related to those earlier symptoms.

As discussed in Chapter Two, many fairly common diseases, including strep throat and mononucleosis, may leave you immunologically vulnerable for future problems. You probably now appreciate the importance of going through your medical history. Any disease, no matter how commonplace, may be a precursor to your present bladder problems.

You should also record all the surgery you have had. Which tissues were removed? Many times I see patients who complain of pain in their lower abdominal right quadrant. It could be a number of things, including an ovarian cyst or appendicitis. Some of these patients have had an ovary removed but don't remember if it was the right one or the left one. They may remember what hospital they were in but not the name of their doctor.

It is simple to obtain the records of any past operations by calling the hospital records office. Your doctors, too, will release your medical records if you sign a consent form requesting it. Keep copies for your own records.

In studying the evolution of your disease, take note of how medicines, especially antibiotics, affected your symptoms. When treated with antibiotics, did your symptoms abate after one or two days or not until a week or ten days later? Were your symptoms better or worse? Did you become allergic to any of the medications?

The idea of evolution forces you to organize your medical history sequentially, not randomly. Follow the process through as you've experienced it. It may help to use birthdates, anniversaries, jobs held, or schools attended as points of reference to recall facts and developments.

Each person's medical evolution is unique. No one can figure it out for you and only you can organize it properly. As we discuss what's happened, I may be able to ask some questions that will remind you of events that you thought were unrelated and that you left out. But we have to work together to get the whole story.

Medications

It's frustrating to have a patient tell me that a doctor gave her a medication, but she doesn't know the name of it. Perhaps all she knows is that it was a little white pill and that it made her sick to her stomach.

Vagueness about medication is ill-advised. Always keep a record of the drugs you take. Either keep the empty prescription bottle or jot down the name of the drug in a little notebook kept in the medicine cabinet. Otherwise, you might get confused.

For example, one woman knew that a purple pill she once took had made her sick. She thought it was Pyridium, a drug sometimes used to treat urinary tract infections, when in fact it was a sulfa drug. When she was later prescribed a sulfa drug for a bladder infection—because she said she was allergic to Pyridium—she got sick!

If you don't know the name of a medicine you've taken, call the doctor who prescribed it for you and ask the nurse to check your medical records. Always keep an up-to-date list of any allergies you have. If a medication gives you unwanted side effects, let all your physicians know about it. Keep everyone who treats you aware of any changes in your body's reactions to drugs and medicines.

We need to know the names of all the medications you take for any health problem. Medicines are excreted in urine and hence may affect bladder tissue, causing urinary tract problems. For example, some antidepressants can keep the bladder muscle from working properly. Medications that relax the intestinal muscles for people with colitis may also cause the bladder muscle to relax and not empty completely.

Keep a record of the exact dosage of all your medications. I know of a woman who didn't realize she was taking an estrogen supplement. As part of the therapy for a bladder problem, a different physician prescribed estrogen therapy. For several weeks, the woman took a double dose of estrogen. She was unharmed but the mistake could have been avoided had she been aware of what was in her pills.

What medicines had no effect? I may be ruminating in the back of my mind about one drug over another to try on you. But if you can tell me that a certain drug previously had no effect, it can save us both time and save you prolonged discomfort.

Combinations of medicines can have untoward effects. Every time a patient tells me she is taking medications that I am not familiar with, I look up the drugs in a reference book and read about all possible drug interactions. Drug interactions do cause urinary tract problems.

For example, Mary Jo regularly took decongestants for her allergies. Later she developed a bladder problem and needed bethanechol chloride to help her void efficiently. The bethanechol chloride stimulated her bladder muscle. But the decongestant tended to close her bladder neck, affecting tissue there much the same way it affected tissue in her bronchial tree. The interaction of bethanechol chloride and decongestant made voiding difficult for Mary Jo. She developed hesitancy and was unable to get her urine stream started while on both medications.

If you take many different medications, I recommend that you go to the library and check out books on prescription drugs and drug interactions. You might want to buy one for home reference. Ask your physicians about drug interactions. It's better to be safe than sorry.

Also, keep a record of the side effects of drugs. Some side

effects can be beneficial. I prescribe an anti-seasickness drug (transderm scopolamine) because, as a side effect, it inhibits bladder contractions and spasms in interstitial cystitis patients. Side effects in general are the price you pay to restore your body's health. They include headache, dizziness, nausea, and tiredness. Some side effects can be avoided by switching medications.

Have you tried home remedies for your urinary problems? It's important to let your physician know everything you're taking, including vitamin pills. Many times I see patients with highly alkaline urine and discover they consume large quantities of calcium carbonate, a calcium supplement for postmenopausal women. All home remedies, including cranberry juice and herbal teas, could potentially contribute to your symptoms. If you have a urothelial membrane leak, acidifying your urine may increase your pain and discomfort. Over-the-counter drugs that you take for colds, allergies, or other common ailments could also be implicated. Take time to make your lists and don't leave anything out.

Associated Problems

Family diseases and other medical problems interrelate in ways that patients never suspect.

Whenever a new patient comes to my office for an evaluation of cystitis, I always ask if she has lower back problems. I'm often greeted with a look of utter surprise, as if I were a Houdini who X-rayed her spine with my eyes. Most women never correlate lower back problems with bladder dysfunction. And, although the correlation between the nerves in the lower back and nerves in the bladder is well-known in urology, many physicians fail to make the association, especially in younger women. But relatively minor back stress, along with other factors, is frequently enough to cause cystitis.

You should know your family's medical history. Are there cases of heart disease, cholesterol problems, diabetes, kidney disease, or anatomic problems with the urinary tract? While interstitial cystitis is an environmental disease, caused by external factors rather than inborn biologic factors, a genetic factor may be involved. I have treated a mother and daughter with interstitial cystitis as well as a daughter and father with the disease.

Many inheritable diseases can interact with the urinary tract. Diabetes is a classic example. Because a diabetic often loses sensory perception, her bladder may lose the ability to sense when it is full. The bladder enlarges and eventually loses the ability to contract and empty properly. Leftover urine promotes the onset of infections.

A diabetic whose disease is not controlled also experiences insatiable thirst. As she drinks more, her bladder walls stretch and the muscle tone deteriorates. I have a patient who develops severe voiding problems every time her insulin fails to manage her diabetes. The rest of the time, her bladder functions normally.

Gout, which involves a buildup of uric acid in the body, is hereditary. It can lead to a class of kidney stones that are difficult to detect by a single radiographic X-ray. This condition requires an intravenous pyelogram (IVP), which is described in Appendix D.

What is your family's cancer history? There is increasing evidence that some families may be prone to a particular type of cancer which may be the result of genetic deficiencies in tissue growth and protective layering.

What are your other medical conditions. Do you have colitis, arthritis, or neurologic problems? Asthmatics often take medications that can affect the bladder and prevent efficient voiding.

When you were treated for an earlier disease, did your doctor prove the diagnosis or only surmise the problem? For example, some patients diagnosed as having pelvic inflammatory disease (PID) have no positive cultures. These patients may have interstitial cystitis. Patients said to have endometriosis likewise may never have had a laparoscopic examination to confirm the gynecologic suspicion of this problem. Many women are told they have a gynecologic problem when in fact it is urologic. And vice versa. The point is that *diagnostic proof should not be ignored.*

I have a patient who was told for two years that she had a chronic uterine infection. But cultures of her urine and cultures of her vagina proved she had no infection at all. Rather, she had interstitial cystitis and went untreated because of poor diagnostic work. If your physician says he has the impression you are suffering from X, Y, or Z, ask, "How do we go about proving that is the problem? What do you recommend to prove a diagnosis?" Laparoscopy proves endometriosis. A positive urine culture proves cystitis. And so on. Be sure your physician treats you for a *real* condition and not for a *probable* cause of your symptoms.

Lab Work

How many times have you been X-rayed? What did those X-rays show? Unless you have records of your laboratory tests, you may forget important findings. People tend to misinterpret or misrelate facts told them about such tests. For example, one person told me her white count was low. In fact, when we got the test records, it was normal. A different blood measure had been low.

Lab tests are useful for determining when a disease process may have begun. Again, test records are available from hospitals, clinics, or the doctors who ordered them. If, for any reason, a physician refuses to release your medical records you can get the records from other sources. It is your legal right to have copies of all your medical records. Personally bring them to the new doctor's office. Don't mail them ahead of time for they might get lost.

Some tests need to be done only once. Avoiding unnecessary repetition of tests saves you time, money, and discomfort. For example, many cystitis patients undergo an IVP, an X-ray study that shows the kidney anatomy and bladder placement (see Appendix D). Once this test result is normal, it rarely needs repeating; people certainly don't need several IVPs as one might need an annual chest X-ray. Moreover, people who are allergic to shellfish should not have an IVP done, since they are likely to be allergic to the iodine used in the procedure. Frequent exposure to radiation in reproductive females should be avoided unless absolutely warranted.

Other tests, such as uroflows and urine cultures, might need to be repeated often, as they reflect current functional status. It all depends on the individual's problems. But not knowing what's been done to you in the past makes it hard for the physician to understand the present and difficult to assess the future.

Emotion

Emotion has been the undoing of women through the ages. It is what makes some women with valid debilitating urologic disease end up in psychiatric hospitals being treated for what is considered an imaginary disease.

The plain fact is that most physicians do not deal well with emotional females.

I have less of a problem getting my women patients to focus on facts because emotion is something that I live with every day. But to many of my male colleagues, an emotional woman is a complete enigma. She is "hysterical" and her complaints make no sense. This has been particularly true of stubborn and, until recently, seemingly causeless and mysterious problems of the female urinary tract.

In my experience, men tend to speak from fact, women tend to speak from emotion. When you tell me that the pain in your bladder is ruining your marriage and destroying your life, you are not giving me factual detail about the pain in your bladder; you are telling me the effects of the problem, not helping me get to the root of it.

THE SAME STORY TOLD TWO WAYS

To show you what I mean, here is the way two women related their symptoms of urinary incontinence during an office visit:

Pateint A: "Dr. Gillepsie, my problem first seemed to begin after I had my second child. I noticed I was having problems controlling the urine but it was not so bad. I only needed to wear a small protective pad when we went out in the evenings. When I was at home, I could usually put my hands between my legs or quickly cross my legs if I was going to sneeze or cough. But lately things have been getting worse. Now that I'm back working again, I find I can't manage the problem the same way. I don't have to get up at night, but one time I did have some pain and burning. I had to get up three or four times. I went to my gynecologist and got a urine culture. It was positive and I was treated with Distaclor; Ceclor (Aust.) for three days. The burning problem went away but I'm still left with the leakage. I'd like to know what can be done."

Patient B: "Dr. Gillespie, I just don't know what I'm going to do in a situation like this anymore. I can't go to my friends' houses anymore. All my friends are sort of staying away from me. I think it's because I ruined my best friend's dining room chair when we were playing cards. When I laughed at a story, before I knew what happened there was a wet spot on the chair. I could feel it on the back of my dress. Well, I really didn't know what to do. I never got asked back. I'm having to wear four or five pads during the daytime and I'm so isolated. I don't know what to do about it anymore."

Patient A gave me accurate, helpful facts without emotion. She knew when she leaked, how much, and what could arrest it. The impact on her life is clear, but the emotion does not cloud or distort the facts. As a physician, I would easily know in what direction to proceed to help this patient.

Patient B has not given me helpful facts. I've heard everything except the kinds of observations that would help in making a diagnosis. Not only did she waste some of our time, but she failed to give me any accurate evidence of her problem other than the fact that she leaks urine when she laughs and she has to wear pads. Evidently she wanted help because her incontinence was ruining her social life.

It may be very hard to separate emotion from observed fact, particularly if you've been to numerous doctors, all of whom failed to find a reason for your symptoms. But don't feel as if no one will ever listen to you.

Many sufferers of chronic cystitis have this outlook on their visits to new physicians. But you need to take each visit with an open mind. If you don't get satisfaction at one place, go to another. An astonishing number of people today are well informed about medicine. Doctors are finding that if they don't give straight answers, the smart medical consumer will take his or her business elsewhere. You don't need to stay with a physician who promotes ignorance, won't explain side effects, or keeps you overmedicated as a way to keep you quiet.

Be aware, however, that chronic pain affects emotional stability. You "trigger" more easily than you would if you were pain-free. Pain makes you more sensitive and unable to tolerate suggestions or inferences—which may be relatively benign. Try not to respond to a physician's questions in a way that infers your problem is psychiatric or emotional.

I sympathize with your agony and pain, but we must concentrate on the factual elements if I am going to help you. Women with interstitial cystitis, for example, live day to day with a kind of unrelenting torture. When they try to relate their symptoms to physicians, understandably they typically focus on their mental anguish. Many physicians then diagnose these women as having a psychosomatic disorder. Thus many women do not get the kind of rational medical treatment more readily given to male patients.

But, as I've stated, women tend to be extremely accurate observers of fact and can use that skill to advantage in their health care. When preparing for your next visit to a doctor, remember the acronym "FEMALE." If you relate facts before emotion, your observations will help to establish a valid interaction with the physician.

FIVE

Anatomy Is *Not* Destiny

A model of the female urinary tract sits on my office desk. It takes up space, gets in my way, and I knock it over from time to time. But for one very important reason it has never left my desk in the six years that I have practiced urology: Most women do not know what their urogenital system looks like. If a picture is worth a thousand words, a model is worth a novel.

To overcome cystitis, you must have a mental picture of how you are built. And so, as part of getting you started on the road to understanding, I am going to discuss your anatomy in the same way as I would sitting with a patient in my office.

Believe it or not, knowledge of the female lower urinary tract is still evolving. Many earlier assumptions about the way women are constructed have been overturned in recent years. Please remember that urology, like other medical specialties, is a fast-moving discipline in which exciting discoveries and new treatments arrive on the scene virtually every month. Our knowledge is not static and even information about basic human anatomy can change.

Your urinary tract is exquisitely adapted for bearing children. Its primary function—the elimination of the body's liquid wastes—is usually carried out effectively and efficiently.

If you encounter problems with your bladder or urinary tract, you may unwittingly be altering nature's design. You may do things or introduce agents that interfere with normal function.

Why Women and Men Must Be Treated Differently

Because men's and women's urinary tracts share the same primary function, the transportation of urine, they often are analyzed according to common assumptions and principles. Naturally all urologists recognize that men and women are anatomically different, but in the final analysis of what can go wrong with the urinary tract, the similarities between men and women often have been held to be more important than the differences.

But the differences are significant (see illustration). The male urinary tract serves a major sexual function while the female tract serves but a secondary sexual function.

Consider the male urethra. As a rule, it measures ten inches from the bladder to the tip of the penis. Its job is to carry urine but also to transport semen during sexual activity. Concepts of physics tell us that the best way to transport a liquid is to move it through a round, smooth channel that holds its shape. The male urethra is ideally designed for this purpose.

The female urethra measures about two inches from the bladder to its opening just below the clitoris. Its primary job is to

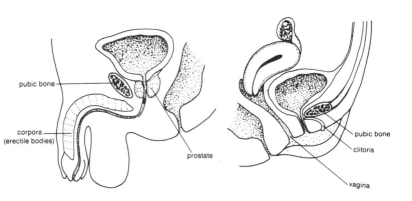

Figure 5-1, Male and Female Anatomy

transport urine. Its sexual role, moving out of the way during childbirth, is secondary. Thus the female urethra is a corrugated tube with a large surface area that can stretch and flatten out when it needs to.

"The Rape of the Female Urethra"

The female urethra has a different, evolutionary function from the male urethra and needs to be studied, examined, and treated differently. When it is not, the consequences can be painful.

For example, the male urethra has a well-defined external sphincter located in front of the prostate gland. The sphincter is a muscle whose job is to close and open like the on-off valve of a garden hose. When open, fluid passes and when closed, fluid cannot pass. The muscle is under somewhat voluntary control.

Unfortunately for men, their urethras are easily infected by certain bacteria, such as gonorrhea. When this happens, scar tissue—called a stricture—forms. The stricture prevents a man from urinating freely. The solution is to dilate or rupture the scar tissue by inserting gradually larger metal rods into the urethra. As you can imagine, this procedure can be very painful.

For decades, some urologists have viewed and treated the female urethra as essentially a shortened version of the male urethra. In this view, challenged only recently, women would also be subject to bacterial infections that create strictures in their urethras. Although women do not get gonorrheal urethritis that causes scarring, they do suffer other bacterial invasions. Thus a common treatment is to stretch open the female urethra to free it of so-called strictures.

Unfortunately, what urologists have been breaking open in women is not a stricture. It is the female external sphincter, which many physicians believed women did not have. As a result, normal tissue is needlessly traumatized and often scarred. The practice is what many urologists now term "the rape of the female urethra."

How Could It Happen?

How could we have not known? One reason is that if you compare the male and female urethras, centimeter per centimeter, it appears that the female sphincter *is* missing. The urethra is not long enough to contain the external sphincter at the same site (see illustration).

But women do have an external sphincter in the urethra. It is a muscle within the wall of the urethra itself, but many urologists believed it to be a birth defect marked by a lack of growth as a woman matured, which supposedly resulted in poor flow and infections in adulthood. Unfortunately, urologists only saw women with infections and never had healthy women in their offices for comparison. All women have this muscle; it is not a birth defect.

Female children found to have bladder infections were frequently diagnosed as having birth defects. Their sphincters were then ruptured by dilation.

Adult women were said to have the child urethral syndrome. Unfortunately, the urethra is frequently blamed for the problems caused by a bladder muscle that does not function properly, often due to back problems that need to be investigated (see Chapter One). If your doctor insists you need a urethral dilation, I advise you to ask for further evaluation, including a uroflow. If the doctor still insists, you might want to get a second opinion.

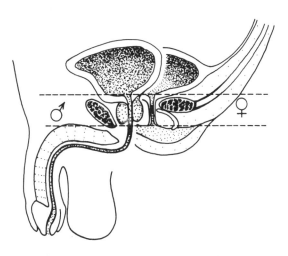

Figure 5-2, Comparing the External Sphincter in Men and Women

It should be noted that in a very few children there is a type of abnormal tissue called a *Lyon's ring*. It may cause infection and reflux. When the ring is dilated, the infection stops. But this is a rare condition and can be picked up with an X-ray. As such, it rarely persists into adulthood.

Women also have some voluntary control over this external sphincter. When you tighten this muscle, you can feel it pull up through the vagina. You can consciously keep the sphincter closed, even when your bladder is uncomfortably full, until you are ready to urinate.

About the only thing that can go wrong anatomically with the female urethra is rare. In developing countries, where some women deliver babies that are too large for their birth canals, the urethra can be ruptured. This rarely occurs in developed nations and should not cause you concern.

More Comparisons and More Differences

Again, comparing men and women, both sexes have glands in the urethra that put out wetting agents to reduce surface tension and let urine pass smoothly over the tissue. These identical glands—called *Skene's glands* in women and *Cowper's glands* in men—are located in pairs at the opening of the female urethra. *Littre's glands,* which also lubricate, are found within the urethra itself. Men alone have the *prostate gland. Prostate* means "guardian." Located below the bladder, it is the gateway through which sperm enter the urethra. It also produces fluids for semen.

Another belief stemming from the comparison of men and women is that the female urethra can be in the wrong place, that it may be too high or too low. There is a birth defect called *hypospadias* that is much more common in men than women. In men, the urethra may not reach the tip of the penis. In this case, it must be surgically extended to restore normal appearance and the flow of urine. In female hypospadias patients, the urethra does not grow long enough and it opens into the vagina. This, too, can be surgically corrected.

Unfortunately, some urologists have taken this concept of a misplaced urethra and extended it to healthy women. The idea is that recurrent infections are promoted or exacerbated by a uretheral opening that is too high or too low. The urethra, they say, is dragged into the vagina with intercourse and this increases bacterial infection. It is "too low" and needs to be raised surgically up out of the vagina. This doesn't make sense. If you can see your urethra on the outside, it's in just the right place.

In all women, the urethra is in the same place—just below the clitoris and above the vagina. Since these openings share common tissue, it is unlikely for them to be in the wrong place. Nevertheless, physicians have surgically cut and repositioned urethras in the hope of stopping infections.

The Bladder Neck

Moving up the urinary tract, features become identical, functionally and anatomically, in men and women. First is the *bladder neck,* located at the bottom or opening of the bladder. *Neck* in this sense means small opening, like the part of a balloon that is tied off. The bladder neck is also called an *internal sphincter.* It, too, is composed of tiny muscles that open and contract like the pupil of an eye.

Your bladder neck serves as the first lock for keeping urine in your bladder. It is not under voluntary control—that is, you cannot consciously cause it to open or close. When a woman's bladder neck is injured, urine can leak out after a cough or sneeze if the external sphincter is not strong enough. However, if she increases her pelvic floor tone by contracting her buttock muscles, she can tightly close the external sphincter to prevent urine from leaking all the way out.

These sphincters—and indeed the entire urinary tract—are laced with networks of nerves that control their action. Nerves leading from your brain are connected to your urinary tract along networks that arrive, via the lower back, at your bladder. One set controls the external sphincter, another the internal sphincter, and others lead to the bladder itself.

These nerves are important to your urologic health, and we will come back to them later.

The Bladder and How It Works

Your bladder, which can be viewed simply as a bag for holding urine, also contains a main sensory area, rich with nerves, that

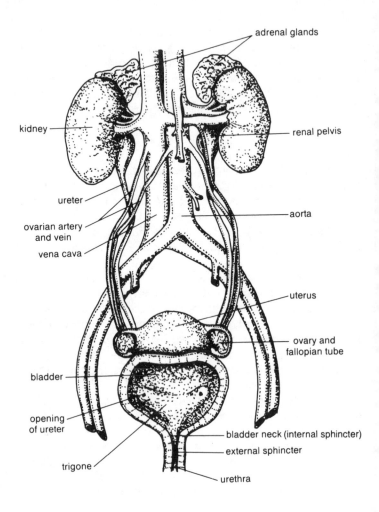

Figure 5-3, The Complete Female Urinary System

signals you when it is time to urinate. Called the *trigone* of the bladder, because of its roughly triangular shape, its tissues derive from a different group of parent cells in the developing embryo than do the tissues in the rest of the bladder. The trigone is special. It is the "signal to void" area of the bladder and its message must be heeded.

The *bladder* itself is like a balloon. Somewhat Y-shaped when empty and spherical when full, it holds a maximum of between twelve and sixteen ounces of urine. In general, comfortable voiding volumes are half this. For reasons as yet unknown, female bladders tend to have larger capacities than male bladders.

The outer part of the bladder is covered with a membrane lining found throughout the abdominal cavity. The bottom is supported by the floor of the bony pelvis. In front, the space between the pubic bones and bladder is filled with loose, fatty tissue. And at the top of the bladder, a strong fibrous cord connects the bladder with the navel.

In order to empty, your bladder must force out fluid, so it is endowed with strong muscular tissue, called the *detrusor,* within its walls. The detrusor must generate enough pressure to cause complete emptying. When it is activated, urine is forced out of the bladder.

Nerves to this muscle also arrive from the lower back. You could compare them to battery cables in your car. These nerves conduct an electrical current to the bladder and stimulate a contraction.

The inside of the bladder, as well as the urethra, is covered with a lining of what are called *urothelial cells*. This lining is protected by a mucous layer that prevents the tissue from being burned by the acid contents of urine. *The GAG layer,* as discussed in Chapter Two, acts as a wetting agent that keeps the lining smooth so that it will be an effective fouling barrier against the acid elements in urine.

The Ureters: Elegant Channels to the Bladder

Urine comes into your bladder through two strawlike structures called *ureters*. About twelve to fourteen inches long, these tubular structures go straight up to your kidneys. Your ureters enter the bladder near its bottom on either side of the trigonal sensory region.

Ureters are simply urine transport channels, but they move liquid in an elegant fashion. It is important that urine cannot move back up into your kidneys, even when you stand on your head. The backward flow of urine can cause damage to kidney tissue by overdistension and by transporting bacteria from the lower urinary tract. This can result in pyelonephritis.

To ensure that fluid moves in only one direction, your ureters make use of special clamplike muscles that contract in waves. Tiny amounts of urine are propelled ever downward by the undulating muscles. A stream of urine spurts into your bladder every ten to thirty seconds. At the entrance to your bladder, again there are strong muscles that prevent urine from going in the wrong direction. At the point where they enter the bladder, the ureters become somewhat thinner, enabling them to collapse and close off as bladder pressures rise.

The Kidneys: Your Purification Machines

Your ureters enter each *kidney* (see illustration) in twin structures that resemble the cup of a lily. This area is, in fact, called the *calyx,* which is Greek for the cup of a flower. The calyx is a boundary region between your kidney and ureter. You can think of it simply as a funnel. There is a junction between the bottom of the funnel (the opening to the ureter) and the region above (the top of the funnel) for collecting liquid.

Urine rolls through a catchment area composed of lots of little cuplike structures. There the urine is finally captured and drained away.

One of your body's vital organs, the kidney delivers all urine to the catchment area. Luckily, we are each born with two kidneys. If one is damaged, we can survive with the other.

Your kidneys serve as the body's purification machine. Your body works much like a factory. You take in "raw materials" (food and drink) and from them extract energy and materials to build the products your body needs. This process creates wastes. Solid wastes are excreted through the colon while liquid wastes are carried through the bloodstream until they can be removed.

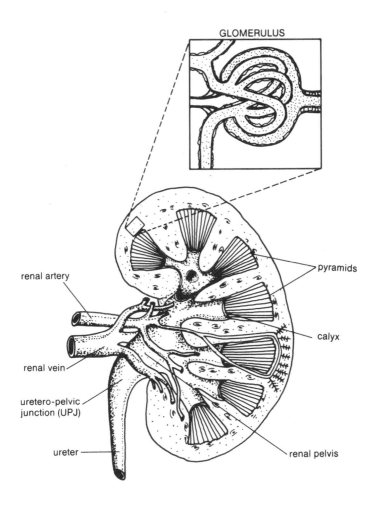

GLOMERULUS

renal artery

pyramids

renal vein

calyx

uretero-pelvic
junction (UPJ)

ureter

renal pelvis

Figure 5-4, A Normal Kidney and Its Small Filtering Units

Your kidneys filter such wastes from blood. They are incredibly efficient filtration devices that extract toxins, acids, and other undesirable products small enough to be carried away in the blood.

Kidneys also maintain a constant volume of blood circulating through your body, regulate fluid balance, control pressure relationships between blood and tissue, and maintain the body's electrolyte system—the relative amounts of sodium, potassium, and water required by every cell in your body.

Every twenty-four hours, the kidneys filter more than forty-five gallons of blood plasma. Most of the materials carried in the plasma can be reused. The kidney's small filters, called *glomeruli,* take out such materials and then return them, in perfect balance, to the circulatory system. About 1 percent of the forty-five gallons that are filtered daily—1.6 quarts—is removed as waste, or urine.

Your urine should be somewhere between pale and darkened yellow, and clear enough so you could read a newspaper through it.

How Much Water Should I Drink?

The volume of urine produced in a day, of course, depends on your environment. In hot, dry climates, a certain amount of your body's liquids is eliminated as perspiration. The wastes are then concentrated in a smaller amount of water. The idea that you should drink eight or more glasses of water a day makes little sense in view of this regulatory mechanism. You should drink as much as feels comfortable, given your level of activity, climate, and diet. Use common sense. On an average, we need thirty-two ounces of fluid a day.

Each kidney is shaped like a bean and measures four and a half inches long, two inches wide, and one to two inches thick. They are located on either side of your spine in the middle of your back and above your waist, under the shoulder blades (see illustration). If you feel pain in your lower back, it is not a kidney infection. The top of each kidney is in fact attached by strong fibers to the diaphragm, and both kidneys rise and fall somewhat as you breathe. Blood is delivered to the kidney by *renal arteries*. (*Renal* just means "pertaining to the kidney.")

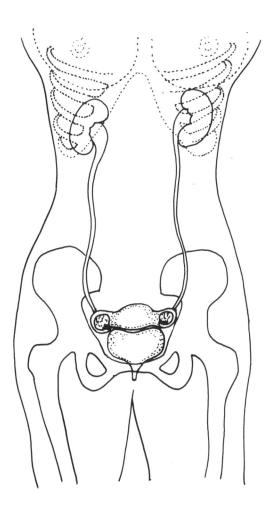

Figure 5-5, The Normal Position of Kidneys

Each kidney has, at a minimum, one million glomeruli, or tiny filtration units. They are the result of one of nature's finest designs.

A Run Through the System

Now let's run through the system from the top down. Suppose you drink a glass of water. It is absorbed into the bloodstream, where it performs numerous jobs before reaching the kidney as a constituent of plasma. Some of the water is extracted as urine and drips, as dew cascades among leaves, down a lubricated pathway to the top of the funnel, or renal pelvis.

When this area collects about a quarter of an ounce of urine, the ureteropelvic junction opens and the urine is propelled down the ureter, in wavelike contractions, to your bladder. A second valve opens and the thimbleful of urine is pushed into the bladder near the trigone area.

Slowly, in this way, your bladder fills from bottom up.

When it is about half full, the trigone begins to stretch under the weight of the accumulating urine. The urine also sends signals to special nerves in the bladder lining. These events signal your brain that you need to consider allowing time to get to an appropriate place to void.

A very complicated, integrated series of functions follows. When you are ready to go, the bladder muscle begins to generate an increase in pressure. As a result, the bladder neck opens and the external sphincter shuts down any activity. You relax your pelvic floor and the bladder muscle contracts. As this happens, the trigone contracts so that your ureters are shut tight, and no urine can flow the wrong way despite the head of pressure.

Voiding is an act of changing pressure gradients. Continence, or staying dry, is the result of the pressure in the urethra being greater than the pressure in the bladder.

The urethra generates its own pressure, which can be measured with instruments. Let's say, on average, it measures "4" on a pressure scale.

The bladder fills passively. As it fills, it does not generate any pressure of its own. Once the bladder is full, however, it does begin to exert pressure which typically, on the same scale, may measure 30. Voiding or urinating occurs when bladder pressure is greater than pressure in the urethra.

As you urinate, pressure in the bladder steadily falls: It goes from 30 to 29, 28, 27, and so on, down to 10, 9, 8, and on down to 5, 4, 3. . . . When it falls below the urethra's pressure—to below 4 on our pressure scale—the urethra's pressure dominates once more. The sphincters close. You stop voiding and, slowly, passively, your bladder begins to fill up again.

You may have noticed that if you hold urine for a very long time, against pressures that can really hurt, you may have trouble, when you finally do go, emptying your bladder completely or voiding with a good, forceful stream. Small amounts of urine may continue to dribble out for a while. This is because you have distended your bladder and it cannot generate its normal pressure head. If you blow up a balloon a second time, making it bigger than it was, the balloon loses elasticity. Your bladder operates under similar principles.

Kidney Malformations and Diseases

Some congenital kidney problems are serious and some are not. I find it fascinating whenever a patient comes in and says, "I have been followed for years by my other doctor for my traveling kidneys." I try not to laugh and ask, "Oh? Where did they book a ticket?" Or, "How far have your kidneys traveled this year?"

The look on the patient's face is quite interesting as I then explain that "traveling kidneys" are normal. The top of each kidney is attached by strong fibers to the diaphragm, so that the kidneys rise and fall during breathing. Some rise and fall, or "travel," more than others. It used to be that surgeons would operate to reposition a traveling kidney. That operation is no longer in vogue because now we know that the position of the kidney has no bearing on its function. If you're told you have a traveling kidney, don't worry. It won't leave you.

An unusual birth defect is the *horseshoe kidney*. During fetal development, both kidneys fail to rise up to their proper place under the rib cage. They lie, like a horseshoe, in the pelvic cavity. Fortunately, the condition rarely bothers its owner; despite the odd placement, the kidneys work fine.

Another birth defect is the *solitary kidney*. One kidney fails to develop and the other, or solitary one, acts as a kind of super kidney. The main drawback of this arrangement is that the owner does not have the protection of two kidneys in case the one is damaged.

An inherited disorder called *polycystic kidneys* can slowly destroy both kidneys. For reasons unknown, numerous small cysts develop in the kidneys and hold urine, as in little sacs. The kidney tissue is ultimately destroyed.

Yet another kidney disease, *fibromuscular hyperplasia,* is more prevalent in women than in men. In this disorder, the main artery going to the kidney takes on the appearance of a string of beads. Blood flow is impeded. As kidney function is impaired, the patient tends to develop high blood pressure. The condition can be corrected by placing a balloon catheter through the artery, thus opening it up and restoring normal blood flow.

Diabetes is probably the best-known kidney disease. With this condition, in which insulin is not taken up properly in the body, excess glucose is circulated in the bloodstream. As the kidneys clear and filter blood, the extra glucose is dumped into urine. In this process, tiny capillaries in the kidneys may eventually become scarred and damaged. Ultimately, the kidneys may lose their ability to properly clear toxins and other substances from the bloodstream.

Another well-known problem is kidney stone disease. Stones may develop in women who repeatedly dehydrate themselves by jogging and other exercise. Dehydration promotes the formation of tiny crystals in the kidney which later pass through the ureters. Other people may develop stones as a result of abnormalities of the parathyroid. Finally, as will be discussed in Chapter Eight, it is not uncommon for stones to pass in some women six weeks or so after childbirth.

Urologists, by the way, have long violated the Hippocratic oath when it comes to dealing with stones. Hippocrates said, "Never cut for stones." Yet, up until very recently, stone surgery has been a mainstay of urologic practice. A new machine called a lithotriptor, developed in Europe and now appearing in major hospitals in the United States, promises to change forever the ways stones are managed. The lithotriptor uses high-energy shock waves generated outside the body to disintegrate stones inside the body while the patient sits in a tub of warm water. Within a few hours, the resulting stone particles—about the consistency of coarse sand—begin to pass naturally from the urinary tract.

Toward a New Understanding of Women's Bodies

You might think that everything there is to know about human anatomy has already been discovered. But that is not the case. As researchers refine their tools and develop greater understanding of how the body functions, they are discovering new nerve networks and systems.

Urology in particular has been somewhat handicapped by its male-dominated view of the urinary tract, but things are changing for the better. Many urologists, both men and women, are coming to understand how function and design differ between the sexes. The better you understand nature's design, the better you are able to care for your body and know when something has gone awry.

SIX

You Don't Have to Live with Incontinence

Millions of adult Americans—no one is certain how many—suffer some degree of urinary incontinence. That is, they do not have complete control over their bladders. To their never-ending embarrassment, they leak urine.

Incontinence is a common problem, yet you never hear much about it. Talk shows don't deal with the topic. Women's magazines and newspaper health columnists rarely write about it.

To my constant amazement, incontinence remains one of the most taboo subjects in American culture. People are willing to talk about their hemorrhoids, constipation, and sexual dysfunction but they do not, in public or private, talk about their incontinence.

Perhaps we, as a society, are fixated on continence—the ability to stay dry—because of our early toilet training experiences. Children are taught that continence is a virtue. It symbolizes our first encounter with self-control. Continence is so deeply intertwined with our unconscious memories of parental approval and disapproval, perhaps we will never be comfortable with the subject.

As a urologist, however, I can make the claim that incontinence is treatable. There are numerous ways to deal with the problem so that whatever the cause, incontinent adults can become fully functioning adults. The more we talk about incontinence, realizing it is not something to be hidden, the more people will discover the treatment that is best for them.

It is not an insignificant problem. For the elderly, incontinence is a major medical, psychological, and social problem. It has been estimated that nursing homes spend up to $1.5 billion a year coping with incontinence. About 40 percent of all the sanitary pads sold in this country are used for incontinence.

Types of Incontinence

Judy's Story: Urinary Stress Incontinence

Judy is a fifty-six-year-old medical librarian with four grown children. Life is supposed to get easier after your children leave, she told me one day last year, "but for me it got worse." Judy leaked urine whenever she laughed, coughed, or sneezed. Her condition, called *urinary stress incontinence,* caused her to leak urine whenever a "stress," such as a sudden sneeze, took her by surprise. With warning Judy could tighten up the muscles on her pelvic floor and sometimes prevent the leak. But most of the time, she could not.

"The problem first began about twenty years ago," she said. "I thought it was just because of childbirth. Unfortunately, women were just led to believe that this is just one of the things that happen to us. I was told not much could be done."

The problem affected Judy's life. "It was minor when it started, but as time went on, it was very difficult. I couldn't do exercises. I was constantly aware of where the restroom was, but it didn't make any difference. It was very difficult.

"Imagine what it's like walking into the dry cleaner's hoping his wife is on duty because you have to explain that you have urine all over your pants or all over your skirt. You have to tell them it's urine. They use certain stain removers and certain cleaning processes for that.

"This went on year after year and I tried doctor after doctor. But often I was patted on the head and told, 'Well, this is what happens to women when they undergo labor.' "

Urinary stress incontinence is the most common type of incontinence for a very simple reason. More often than not, it is a consequence of childbirth. Given the number of American women who have given birth, naturally it is a widespread problem.

Stress incontinence, like many disorders, follows a continuum. It can be mild or severe or anything in between. It usually develops slowly in women ten years or so after they have finished having children.

As a baby moves down the vaginal canal during birth, its head lodges underneath the bladder neck. It rests there temporarily before final expulsion through the vagina. If the baby stays in this position for very long—perhaps because its head is big for the mother—stress is imposed on the ligaments that support the bladder neck.

By and large, this stress has no immediate consequences. A few women experience more severe compression to nerves in the vaginal canal and are unable to void twenty-four hours after delivery. Permanent damage is rare, however, and most women quickly resume normal urinary function.

But years later, once gravity begins to affect muscular tone, the bladder neck may slowly start to descend into the vaginal canal. As it does so, it pulls along a small portion of the bladder and forms a protrusion called a *cystocele*. A cystocele holds urine. When you void, your bladder does not empty totally at once because there is always a little bit of urine resting in the cystocele. You have a fallen or dropped bladder.

HOW TO TELL

You can tell if you have a cystocele if you put your fingers in your vagina and then purposely cough or strain. If something comes down and touches your fingers near the opening of your vagina, you have a cystocele.

Another way to tell is by noticing how you void. If you wait a moment and another little squirt of urine always comes out, you probably have a cystocele. That little squirt is the cystocele emptying.

Cystocele means "bladder hernia." It is simply a saclike protrusion of bladder tissue that isn't located higher up, where it belongs. When a cystocele holds urine, the weight of the urine tends to tug on the bladder neck. Under this strain, the bladder neck is unable to generate its normal closing pressure.

When you laugh unexpectedly, sneeze, or run in place, a shock wave is sent through the bladder neck. A normal bladder stays closed under such everyday stress. But a bladder neck weakened by childbirth and pulled upon by a cystocele just opens up. You leak.

When a person with stress incontinence has forewarning, say, that a sneeze is coming, she can sometimes prevent urine from leaking by clamping down consciously on her external sphincter in the urethra. But when there is no warning, which is most of the time, she leaks.

Many women with this problem practice what are called Kegel exercises to strengthen the muscles in the pelvic floor. These isometric exercises are simple to do. Feel your buttock muscles tighten and relax as you pull up and inward with your vagina. I recommend that women do them every day while they brush their teeth. That rolls two habits into one. With improved muscle tone, a woman who sneezes can exert enough external pressure on her urethra to prevent urine from leaking out.

I'm convinced that women who have very rapid baby deliveries and who have very flexible perineums do not generally develop stress incontinence. But those with less flexible perineums, who tend to need episiotomies to help deliver their babies, are candidates for this type of incontinence. Much also depends on how long a fetus's head rests against the bladder neck before the transition stage of labor begins. Of course the number of children borne is also a factor. Many women develop stress incontinence after a third or fourth baby is delivered.

Women with stress incontinence leak different amounts. In my mind, it doesn't matter how much you leak—I don't care whether you wear four maxipads or one minipad each day—at issue is the loss of bladder control. Some urologists will tell you that unless you soak eight pads a day, your problem is not serious enough to fix. I do not concur, because incontinence is treatable, and no one should have to put up with it unnecessarily.

Pity Great-Grandma, for this was not true for past generations and it is still not true for women in many developing countries. When a woman gives birth without medical assistance to a baby that is too large for her body, she may develop tears in her urethra that are called *fistulas*. Forceps deliveries can also traumatize urethral and rectal tissues. Women with fistulas leak urine continuously. The leak may be small or large. Some women must wear adult diapers to accommodate the problem.

There are, however, several surgical techniques available to close and repair fistulas. The tears are carefully layered and stitched in such a way that urine cannot find its way past the sutures.

In past generations, women had to live with fistulas. They devised many techniques for catching urine or for masking its odor. Their techniques became as secretive as the cause of their problem.

Kate's Story: Overflow Incontinence

Kate is a forty-one-year-old account executive at a leading advertising agency in New York. She has a mild case of diabetes that was diagnosed after her daughter was born seven years ago. Kate carefully watches her diet, exercises, and gives herself regular insulin injections. Her diabetes is under control.

But last year, Kate developed a vexing bladder problem. She sometimes found that when she got up from her chair, she had leaked. Other times, she had not. When she bent over to pull on her pantyhose or tie her sneakers, she sometimes leaked. Other times bending over, she did not. Then there were times that she leaked while lying in bed, flat on her back. There was no warning. No sensation of "I have to go now." No pattern to predict when the leaking would occur.

Then, in one month, she developed two bacterial bladder infections, one right after the other. She went to her doctor and got a physical exam. Her insulin levels were correct and her blood sugar was in normal range. But to her great dismay, the surprise leaking continued. What could be causing it?

* * *

Kate suffers from what is called *overflow incontinence*. The name refers to the fact that her bladder muscle is not functioning properly. While it can happen to anyone, it often plagues diabetics or those with severe lower back problems.

Diabetics encounter two problems with their urinary tracts. One is that they lose sensory perception to many nerves, including the nerves that send signals to the bladder muscle. The bladder gets only weak signals that it is time to contract. The second problem is one of overdistension. Diabetics are constantly thirsty when their system is out of balance and they drink copious amounts of water. This causes the bladder muscle to distend and lose tone. Some diabetics' bladders hold twice the normal amount of urine—as much as 1,000 milliliters—because of this stretching.

Imagine Kate's bladder as a bucket that is filled to the top. Because she has lost sensory mechanisms, she can void only with a pressure that empties a quarter of her bladder each time she goes. Her bladder never empties completely and it does not take long for her bladder to overfill. Since she has lost the feeling to know when to void, Kate begins to leak. As her bladder never empties completely, she is susceptible to cystitis. If her blood sugar were not contro led, the resulting high sugar content of her urine would be especially conducive to bacterial growth.

Unlike Elizabeth, who only leaks when she sneezes, coughs, or is otherwise stressed, Kate leaks without any warning. She has a functional problem, not an anatomic problem. Her bladder neck is intact and all the angles of her urinary tract are correct. Thus surgery is the wrong way to correct Kate's problem.

Kate's problem is a weakened bladder and weakened "battery cables" (nerves to her bladder). The first step in treatment is to restore neural transmission through oral doses of synthetic acetylcholine called bethanechol chloride. This drug is a carbon copy of the body's natural chemical transmitter, acetylcholine. Flooding her "battery" (the bladder) with "battery acid" (the drug) strengthened the weak transmission of the charge from her nerves, and her bladder began to empty more efficiently.

In addition to keeping her diabetes under control, Kate put herself on a voiding schedule. At home she wore a small kitchen timer around her neck that rang every two hours. At work she was able to remind herself within other scheduling routines. With time, she regained some of her original bladder tone.

Overflow incontinence also affects people who do not have diabetes. A woman came to my office last year saying she had to wear nine or ten pads on the days she leaked most. Some days were better than others. Most of the time when she leaked, she did not have any warning. She also leaked when she coughed or sneezed.

I asked her about her back. She said she had some small discomfort. An X-ray showed there was compression of her fourth and fifth lumbar vertebrae. Another X-ray study, a voiding cystourethrogram, showed that her bladder neck had lost support. As with many incontinent people, there were multiple aspects to her problem.

I gave her bethanechol chloride to help correct the bladder muscle problem. By augmenting neural transmission to the detrusor, her overflow incontinence was brought under control.

To correct the bladder neck problem, we tried another medication called *ephedrine,* a decongestant that causes the bladder neck to close down.

This patient responded very well to "chemical surgery." She did not undergo corrective anatomic surgery because her problem could be controlled by medications alone. If we had corrected only her neural problems, she would have remained with stress incontinence. If we had surgically repaired her bladder neck, she would have been susceptible to repeated bladder infections because she would still have been unable to empty her bladder.

It is very important that your physician differentiate all the causes of cystitis and incontinence because several problems can occur simultaneously and therefore multiple treatments may be required. The urinary tract is composed of multiple units, and one or more parts can go awry.

Melissa's Story: Urge Incontinence

Melissa has a different kind of problem called *urge incontinence.* The first time she experienced it, she was at the movies.

Halfway through an engrossing film, she realized she had to void. She made her way to the bathroom, only to find a line. The urge to go became greater and greater. Before she could get to a stall, the urine poured out of her and thoroughly wet her clothing.

People with urge incontinence experience strong bladder contractions at unexpected times. The bladder empties of its own accord. If you have a severe bladder infection, for example, you may experience tremendous urgency and spontaneous voiding, as the bladder tries to expel the infected urine. More commonly, the problem tends to be caused by damage to nerves in the upper back, above the fourth and fifth lumbar. Back injuries, strokes, and diseases such as multiple sclerosis can lead to such neural damage.

Voiding/X-rays

This is a photograph of an X-ray of the bladder and bladder neck of a patient with urinary stress incontinence. See the little beaking at the bottom. That's her open bladder neck. When she coughs or sneezes, I can observe the contrast media in the urine going through the bladder neck.

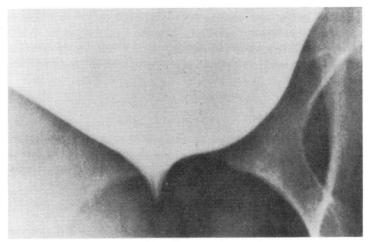

Figure 6-1, Stress Incontinence

As a result, there is a lack of inhibitory fibers that release an enzyme that stops the activity of acetylcholine. Inhibitory signals are blocked and only activating signals get through to the bladder, telling it to contract. Then the urge to urinate is uncontrollable.

This type of incontinence is treated with medications that block acetylcholine transmissions. Pro-Banthine (propantheline bromide) or oxybutynin chloride work by relaxing the bladder muscle, in an attempt to keep it from responding to the excess signals to void.

These are secondary management approaches that treat the symptoms rather than the cause of such incontinence. The cause, in many of these cases, may be a stroke or other brain damage that cannot be corrected. Many times injured backs and damaged discs cannot be repaired. Thus medications are often the best route to controlling such incontinence.

In Melissa's case, she was found to have "writer's neck" caused by vertebral instability that was putting pressure on her spinal column. Surgery relieved this compression and her voiding returned to normal.

Choosing the Right Treatment for Incontinence

If you suffer from incontinence, you need to find out what is causing the problem before you have any treatment done. When incontinence has anatomic causes, surgery may be the answer. When it is caused by a functional problem, medication may be the answer.

Surgical Procedures

There are many surgical procedures to prevent incontinence caused by anatomic problems. Like incontinence itself, these operations run a gamut from uncomplicated to very complicated.

TEFLON ANYONE?

For patients with mild stress incontinence, there is a new and simple technique that can be done in my office. The technique is about ten years old and was first developed in Europe. Teflon, the same material that lines nonstick cookware, is injected directly into tissue to give it added volume. The technique has been used to thicken the vocal cords of people with paralyzed larynxes. Urologists use it to thicken the bladder neck in the same way.

The Teflon treatment is not for everybody. It tends to work on women who have small cystoceles and mild stress incontinence. Women with large cystoceles cannot be helped this way because enough Teflon cannot be packed into the tissue without the added weight of urine pulling open the bladder neck.

Before injecting the Teflon, I anesthetize the urethra with a cotton-tipped swab soaked in a liquid anesthetic. I then place a longer swab with anesthetic up to the bladder neck. All the pain sensation nerves in the urethra, up to the bladder, are then paralyzed. If your doctor knows how to anesthetize the urethra (and unfortunately many do not!), you will feel no discomfort.

While other urologists perform this procedure under general anesthesia, I find that local anesthesia produces more satisfactory results. When I was taught how to do this procedure in Europe, it was always done under general anesthesia. But upon returning to the States and thinking it over, I decided to alter the procedure. When the patient is awake, she can cooperate. By coughing or sneezing, she can help me determine how much Teflon is needed to close off her bladder neck and whether or not we have achieved total continence. I have given Teflon injections in this manner to more than twenty women and all are doing extremely well—better, I think, than if they had not been awake to help.

During the procedure, I pass a cystoscope through the urethra to view the bladder neck. Using a long special needle, I then inject Teflon into the musculature of the bladder neck. The amount varies, depending on each woman's anatomy. The goal is to bring bladder neck tissue together in order to duplicate the normal anatomy of continence.

Once the Teflon is injected, the patient never feels it.

Since the procedure has been around only a few years, we don't yet know how long the treatment will be effective. It could last a lifetime for some women. Others might need small amounts of Teflon added in the future.

This technique is not yet widespread, but by selecting a candidate properly, excellent results can be obtained.

Judy, for example, was an excellent candidate. She was so happy after her surgery, in fact, that she appeared with me on the

"Hour Magazine" television show to tell women all over the country about her experience. How did it change her life?

"It's been a year now and it's just remarkable," Judy told her interviewer. "To have gone from a constant awareness of the possibility of a problem—heavy sanitary pads, be sure to wear cotton clothing if you're going to be gone a long time, always the fear of odor, and so on—is just remarkable. Now I've thrown away all those heavy old things. No problem! Exercise is fine.

"The Teflon procedure is really an amazing thing. There's no pain, no difficulty. When it's over, its sort of like getting up from the table and throwing away your crutches. But I tossed away something else."

Now that aerobic exercise is popular, many women are finding out that they leak when they run in place or do jumping jacks. Some trot off to the bathroom in the middle of the exercise routine while others wear pads. (Running or jumping do not *cause* incontinence. However, such exercise can unmask an anatomic problem that is already there.) The Teflon treatment is well suited to such women who tend to have a mild form of stress incontinence.

A "FACE LIFT" FOR THE BLADDER

When the bladder neck is wide open and the cystocele is what we would term moderate, the success rate for Teflon surgery decreases markedly. If this is your problem, there are other approaches we can take. You may be a candidate for what amounts to a face lift of the bladder.

The goal of this surgery, known as an *anterior repair,* is to tighten the vaginal tissue underneath the bladder. The surgeon, usually a gynecologist, cuts some vaginal tissue and pushes the cystocele back up. He or she then gathers the vaginal tissue, tucking in some of its "wrinkles," and sews it up tightly. This gives more support to the bladder's base so that the bladder neck is often brought back into alignment.

The procedure is designed to correct cystoceles, not to correct major problems of the bladder neck. Patients with large cystoceles but minor bladder neck problems find great success with this surgical approach.

An advantage of this operation is that it leaves no readily visible scars because everything is done through the vagina. However, anterior repairs—like face lifts—may need to be redone after several years.

Keep in mind that your problem may change with time. A cystocele may be controlled while a bladder neck problem worsens. Remember that each part of the urinary tract has many subunits that can fail. Different problems occur at different times.

HOW RECONSTRUCTION TECHNIQUES CAN BRING DRAMATIC IMPROVEMENT

For many people, bladder control is lost because supportive tissue that normally helps close down the bladder neck is out of alignment. With the system askew, there is no pressure available to help close the bladder neck.

The ultimate cause of this problem is gravity. As women age, there is loss of muscle tone in the bladder neck. Because of neurologic damage from pregnancy and childbirth, the bladder neck falls. The aqueduct opens. There is no resistance left in the pipeline to keep the water back inside the dam. Urine flows like water through a pipe whose faucet is stuck open.

Women with this problem tend to have severe incontinence, requiring more than one or two pads a day to maintain dryness. It is for this kind of incontinence that urologists do reconstructive surgical procedures. The idea behind each technique is to create compression and resupport the bladder neck area. By altering pressure gradients, continence can be restored. Continence, if you recall from Chapter Five, occurs when pressure in the urethra is greater than pressure in the bladder.

An early technique, called the *Marshall-Marchetti-Krantz procedure,* was developed by three surgeons to correct incontinence in a man. It was found to work so well in women that it is exclusively used for stress incontinence (which men rarely have).

Unlike the anterior repair, this surgery requires an abdominal incision. The surgeon then sutures the tissue supporting the bladder neck and urethra to the pubic bone for support. This pulls the bladder neck forward, angling it much like a Chinese finger trap. When you cough or sneeze, the pressure flowing from your abdomen is directed into the pubic bone, not down the urethra. With this added support, you stay dry.

However, this procedure requires that you have a well-functioning bladder muscle. If the bladder neck is obstructed but the bladder muscle is not strong enough to empty the bladder, you could trade your incontinence for cystitis. Before undergoing this operation, *it is important to have a uroflow and cystometrogram done to document how well you void.* Patients have to realize that once continence is restored, they may have to fine tune or adjust the system back into balance, much as they do with the color on a television set.

This operation is a major form of surgery that must take place in a hospital. The stay is a week to ten days. The incision is usually made from below the belly button down to the pubic bone. It leaves a longitudinal scar.

As with any surgery, be sure that you choose a physician who is experienced with the procedures and knows when they are indicated and how to select patients for each approach. If you find someone who has performed this operation several times, your operation is likely to have fewer complications.

Another type of operation, with several variations, is done through the vagina. It is called a *Stamey urethropexy* or a *Pereyra procedure.* Unlike the Marshall-Marchetti-Krantz procedure, an incision is made in the vagina. Tissue on both sides of the bladder neck (called the endopelvic fascia) is then grasped and sutures are placed through it. Next, a tiny cut is made just above the pubic bone, along the pubic hair line, and a special instrument is passed through the hole to pick up the sutured material down below the vagina. Like a crochet needle, the instrument pulls the sutures up to the abdominal wall. The sutures are cross-tied for support. You now have a suspension bridge mechanism for supporting the bladder neck.

During surgery, a tube is put through a hole in the lower abdomen in order to drain urine. In this way, a catheter between your legs is eliminated while swelling caused by the operation subsides. By turning the spigot knob on and off, voiding can be practiced and it is easy to tell how much urine is left behind. Once normal voiding resumes, the tube is removed.

This procedure requires only a one-day stay in the hospital and is very successful. I performed this surgery on one of my sisters, which shows what confidence my family has in me. Within a week she was back at work and she never lost a drop!

ARTIFICIAL SPHINCTERS

Some patients have problems that cannot be surgically corrected by any of the methods already described. Certain pelvic injuries and birth defects such as spina bifida can create complicated bladder function problems which would be made worse by a static obstruction procedure. In these patients, using an artificial sphincter to restore continence can be very helpful.

The sphincter (see photograph) is a cuff that is placed around the bladder neck region. A little bulb goes from the cuff down to the labia. A reservoir of fluid sits in the abdomen and controls needed pressure gradients for voiding. Water from the reservoir

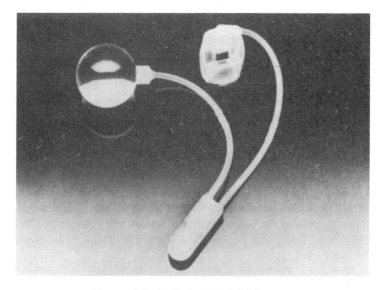

Figure 6-2, AMS Artificial Sphincter

(Courtesy of American Medical Systems, Inc.,
Minnetonka, MN)

flows into the cuff and is maintained there for as long as you want to stay dry. When you want to void, you merely go into the bathroom and squeeze the bulb that is tucked into the labia. The pressure gradient changes and urine flows out of the bladder.

In this way, patients with paralyzed bladder muscles can control their own continence. However, mechanical devices do have mechanical failures. In experienced hands and with good designs, artificial sphincters are successful.

Nonsurgical Procedures: Medicine Only, Please

Many cases of incontinence are not caused by anatomic problems. If your problem is caused by functional or neurologic problems, you should never have surgery without first undergoing a complete urodynamic evaluation.

If lower back injury, diabetes, or any other disease is preventing chemical neurotransmitters from reaching your bladder, you may respond to medicines to correct the deficiency. I prefer to assess what can first be done functionally for a patient. I'm constantly surprised at how effective the right combination of medications can be in restoring continence.

Patients with overflow incontinence, caused by bladder muscle underactivity, may require 100 milligrams of bethanechol chloride a day. That's four 25-milligram pills a day. Someone with urge incontinence may require an antispasmodic medication such as Pro-Banthine at 15 milligrams four times a day.

The two most commonly prescribed drugs for incontinence are bethanechol chloride and Pro-Banthine. One stimulates smooth muscle to contract while the other inhibits it. As you might expect, these medications have opposite side effects.

Bethanechol chloride may cause blood pressure to increase a bit whereas Pro-Banthine may drop blood pressure. Bethanechol chloride may cause some people to sweat and it increases the heart rate. Pro-Banthine dries the mouth and slightly decreases the heart rate.

As with all medications, whether they are blockers or augmenters, you need to modify dosage as therapy progresses. I do this by monitoring the patient's condition with repeat uroflows. If I find that your bladder is generating too much of a contraction, causing you to void too often, the dose of a stimulating drug is too high. In contrast, the dose of an antispasmodic medication may be too high if you are having difficulty in voiding. We then adjust the dose accordingly, which allows you to void more normally.

My goal in treating incontinence and cystitis is to correct the root of the problem. If there is any way we can correct the primary cause, such as through exercises to strengthen back muscles, you will not need to use medications forever. By stabilizing the lower back and relieving pressure on the nerves to the bladder, many women can throw their medications away.

Learning to Adapt

Doris is seventy-two years old, and although she has had many experiences, last year was the most embarrassing time of her life. She has been incontinent for several years now, resulting from a lower back problem and the legacy of childbirth. And like many people her age, Doris is not a good candidate for surgery. She has had to learn to live with incontinence.

But last year took the cake. During her golden wedding anniversary, with all her friends around, she leaked. Every time she got up to dance, the urine spot on the back of her dress grew bigger and bigger. Everyone noticed, but she didn't discover the spot until later and she thought she would die of embarrassment.

When Doris came to me, she was in tears. Some days she was using only two pads, but on other days she needed six. She really didn't care how many pads she had to use. She just didn't want to leak all over her clothes, she wanted to diminish the odor, and she was tired of having her skin burned by urine.

A combination of techniques helps people like Doris. One was devised by another patient who solved part of the problem by designing a half-slip out of plastic that neatly covers the back of her dress or skirt. When she's out to dinner or playing cards with friends, she can laugh and have a good time without worrying that she'll wet the chair. Anyone can fashion such a half-slip, and I guarantee that it works!

To prevent the odors that build up when urine is concentrated, I recommended to Doris that she drink a lot of water. Although she continued to leak, and she had to use more pads, there was less ammonium in her diluted urine, so the odor did not cause further embarrassment.

Many incontinent people are always wet, and their skin becomes leathery from exposure to urine. Such tissue is easily cracked, causing it to bleed. When acid urine comes into contact with such wounds, the pain is indeed terrible. To protect her skin from being burned by urine, Doris began using a cream containing vitamins A and D. Like creams used to protect babies from diaper rash, it provides a molecularly balanced barrier against urine and works to heal ammonia burns.

Doris stopped by to see me several months after we first met. She showed me photographs of her two grandchildren and said that her life was much improved. Using these methods, she was now comfortable in social situations.

* * *

Ten Warning Signs of Bladder Problems

• leakage of urine that prevents desired activities;

• leakage of urine that causes embarrassment;

• leakage of urine that began or continued after an operative procedure (hysterectomy, cesarean section, prostate surgery, lower intestinal or rectal surgery);

• inability to urinate (retention of urine) following an operative procedure;

• urinating more frequently than usual without a proven bladder infection;

• needing to rush to the bathroom and/or losing urine if you do not arrive in time;

• pain related to filling of the bladder and/or pain in relation to urination (in the absence of a bladder infection);

• frequent bladder infections;

• progressive weakness of the urinary stream with or without a feeling of incomplete bladder emptying;

• abnormal urination or changes in urination related to a nervous system abnormality (stroke, spinal cord injury, multiple sclerosis, etc.).

Remember: Incontinence is not a disease. It is a symptom of an underlying condition.

People are starting to demand that something be done about incontinence. But before progress can be made, both patients and doctors need to understand better their obligations in the matter. If you are ashamed to discuss the problem, no one will be able to help you. If doctors think incontinence is hopeless and, God forbid, "incurable," they may fail to help you.

In many instances incontinence cannot be "cured" in the sense that the problem disappears forever. But incontinence can be well managed so that people may lead normal lives. This is certainly better than the alternative of being frightened and lonely, unable to be with friends.

As a urologist, I will do my best to bring the subject of incontinence into the arena of public debate and consciousness. It is a problem that has been overlooked and ignored far too long.

SEVEN

How Menopause and Aging Affect Your Urologic Health

In the Cameroon highlands of West Africa, there lives a sixty-two-year-old grandmother named Mami Estah, whose attitude toward life is most instructive. Until she was fifty, Mami Estah's primary role in life was that of wife and mother. She raised eight children, cooked, tended her farm, and sold extra crops in the market. Her life was dominated by duties and routines.

But when Mami Estah entered menopause, everything changed. She was liberated. She left her husband, bought two cases of beer, and opened a bar. She rented out a back room. As the bar became successful, Mami Estah entered local politics. She became the eyes and ears for friends in the capital and grew so powerful that the prime minister paid her many visits. As was the custom for women of her status, Mami Estah took "wives" to grow her food, cook, and clean for her. The wives took male lovers but the children were "fathered" by Mami Estah. Eventually she ran for office and became powerful in her political party.

In Mami Estah's culture, premenopausal women have very defined roles and little opportunity to move outside prescribed tasks. But once a woman enters menopause, the restrictions are lifted. She is free to operate in society much as a man. With her childbearing years behind her, she can do whatever she pleases.

Somehow, in our supposedly more advanced culture, American women tend to fear that life is finished after the children are gone. The empty nest syndrome strikes. Menopause is not a time of celebration and liberation. It is not perceived as a life passage that brings opportunity and challenge. Instead, many American women become fearful and mournful upon entering menopause. Many fail to plan for this period of their lives and fail to take up new challenges. Mami Estah would certainly pity them.

What is it about menopause that frightens so many of us? The word itself comes from Greek and means "ending of the monthly." Around the age of forty-five or fifty, regular menstrual cycles become increasingly irregular and then stop. Before menopause, we ovulate and are capable of having children. After menopause, we stop ovulating and can no longer have children.

The most significant medical consequence of menopause is loss of estrogen, which can drop by 75 percent. As I have noted, estrogen is related to maturity of the secretions that protect the urinary tract. When, in menopause, estrogen levels decline, the bladder lining and vaginal tissues become more prone to bacterial adherence. The vagina is less elastic. During intercourse, tissue may be abraded. The vagina may contract, actually shrink in size.

While this may sound frightening, you do not need to worry. Our sex lives do not come to an abrupt end at menopause. There are currently more than thirty million postmenopausal women in the United States. Each woman can expect to live about a third of her life, and a full and vibrant third, after menopause.

Nevertheless, modern medicine still has much to learn about the natural biologic transition of menopause. Scientifically speaking, it is a phenomenon full of mysteries. Neither the male nor the female reproductive tract is fully understood. Research about both sexes is active.

The study of the male urogenital tract falls to urologists. That is, we study and treat a man for problems of his reproductive system as well as his urinary tract. But, as far as the medical profession is concerned, women require two kinds of specialist.

Gynecologists study and treat problems of the female reproductive system. Many of them also practice obstetrics, which involves the special needs of pregnancy and childbirth. Urologists, however, treat the woman's urinary tract only; her reproductive system is someone else's business. There is no textbook for urologists on menopause, let alone a chapter on the subject in any urology book.

Because pregnancy and childbirth are complex, it is easy to understand why specialties arose to handle the process. But, in contrast to males, there *is* an overlap between specialties in handling the female urogenital system; urologic and gynecologic problems are not mutually exclusive.

Menopause is primarily a gynecologic event. Yet you would be surprised how many women come to urologists with problems that can be traced to their menopause. Menopause most definitely has urologic implications. On the other hand, many women go to a gynecologist for basic urologic problems, such as incontinence. The point is that your reproductive tract and urinary tract can affect one another. This seems especially true in menopause.

What Happens When Estrogen Levels Drop

Your vagina has a layer of protective coating, the layer that keeps bacteria from adhering to its surface. The coating is dependent on hormones. When you lose estrogen, the coating decreases. You can develop vaginitis (inflammation of the vagina), yeast infections, or vaginal bacterial infections. You may feel itching or urinary frequency.

Such symptoms are sometimes treated with antibiotics. *But this may only worsen the problem*. The vagina possesses a delicate balance of what you might think of as "friendly bacteria." One, called lactobacillus, is known to help prevent harmful bacteria from adhering to tissue. Antibiotics can wipe out the defensive lactobacilli along with any "unfriendly bacteria" that may have caused your infection. In any case, after taking an antibiotic, you need to restore lactobacillus balance as soon as possible.

There are several ways to do this. One is the old home remedy of douching with yogurt. It works because yogurt contains lactobacillus, the same bacteria you need in your vagina. If you find this too messy, you can douche with a special acidophilis-lactobacillus preparation that is sold in health food stores. It does not help, however, to take lactobacillus orally, in products such as acidophilus or raw milk. The human gut digests or destroys these helpful bacteria (which are good for you), but none make it to your vagina through this route. You must add the lactobacilli externally to help your vagina. It works only temporarily and does not restore the lactobacillus to the tissue permanently.

In general, douching is not a good practice. Some women are told to douche to prevent the vaginal odor that sometimes accompanies menopause. But regular douching can dry vaginal tissue, giving bacteria a better surface on which to adhere. Constant douching can even lead to cystitis when vaginal bacteria make their way into the bladder.

Nowadays most gynecologists recommend estrogen replacement therapy to healthy women entering menopause. Since menopause is a gradual process, changes of vaginal tissue can also be gradual. Thus you may start out replacement therapy with an estrogen cream applied directly to the vagina. Later, when estrogen levels have fallen more, you may need oral doses of estrogen. Two hormones, estrogen and progesterone, are often given together.

Estrogen or Estrogen and Progesterone?

Many women are confused about the pros and cons of estrogen therapy versus estrogen/progesterone therapy. And no wonder. Studies show there are dramatic trade-offs. It is a confusing picture.

For example, a highly respected long-term study found that women who took estrogen may have a lower incidence of heart disease than women who took no hormones. Estrogen appears to raise what is termed your body's good cholesterol, which is a factor in preventing heart disease; the implication is that estrogen replacement is good for your heart. Another study showed that estrogen helped prevent osteoporosis, which means it is good for your bones. Indeed, the relationship between osteoporosis and estrogen deficiency has been known for almost half a century.

But other studies have shown that estrogen replacement therapy increases your risk of developing cancer of the uterine lining, called the *endometrium;* the implication is that estrogen replacement is bad for your uterus. Indeed, if you have ever had cancer of the breast or uterus, your physician will most likely not prescribe hormone replacement therapy. Some cancers are estrogen-related and it is prudent not to increase your exposures.

But for healthy women it is a different story. To counteract the risk of endometrial cancer, many physicians about ten years ago began prescribing progesterone along with estrogen. The logic? Since estrogen causes tissue maturation, it builds up the endometrial lining. Progesterone has the opposite effect, causing loss of maturation and breaking down the lining. In other words, progesterone breaks down what estrogen builds up. On the double hormone therapy, you resume menstruation and have regular periods.

The medical profession is divided on the question of hormone replacement therapy. Although evidence strongly suggests that estrogen users are at increased risk for endometrial cancer, the magnitude of that risk is quite low. Endometrial cancer is a rare disease. Estrogen users have the same risk of getting it as do non-estrogen users who are obese. Furthermore, endometrial cancer is a slow-growing cancer with minimal invasion into the uterus. It is usually diagnosed early and survival rates for women with the disease are high. In fact, overall, estrogen-associated cancers do not appear to cause a decrease in life expectancy.

The question remains: Will the double hormone therapy be good for both your heart and your uterus? The answer is not yet clear. People have not been taking the estrogen/progesterone combination long enough for researchers to find the answer. Despite the lack of answers, it is popular today to take progesterone with estrogen to decrease the risk of endometrial cancer.

But I consider the double therapy is similar to taking oral contraceptives and carries similar risks. Progesterone may, in fact, negate the beneficial effects of estrogen and result in a higher health risk (for heart disease, osteoporosis, and strokes) than taking no hormonal therapy at all. Until these issues are clarified, I believe that the use of progesterone is premature.

Hormone Therapy and Urinary Problems

If, like Meryls, you have chronic bladder disease, there is no question that progesterone can be harmful. Merlys is a patient of mine who was treated for interstitial cystitis and remained symptom-free for one year. Then, as she went through menopause, her gynecologist gave her estrogen and progesterone replacement therapy. Her life quickly changed for the worse. Whenever she took the progesterone, Merlys developed cramps, bleeding, and migraine headaches. Her bladder hurt and her urinary pH shot up.

She came to me for help with her bladder. It was clear that the estrogen was increasing cellular maturation in her bladder and helping form the protective layer on the bladder surface. But progesterone was tearing down what estrogen built up. Merlys's bladder was abnormal and it could not tolerate the double hormonal therapy.

Unfortunately, Merlys's doctor refused to give her estrogen only. She said Merlys had to be cycled monthly on progesterone regardless of her bladder problem. And the doctor also refused to acknowledge that the migraine headaches were associated with progesterone (although such a link has been made in several studies.)

Merlys conferred with an endocrinologist (an expert on hormones) and was given a different option. She could take estrogen only, which was good for her vagina and bladder, and if she should develop abnormal bleeding, an endometrial biopsy could easily be performed in the office.

Merlys chose this option and found a new gynecologist who would follow her closely. She tallied all the risks and actively took responsibility for her health.

In general, women with chronic bladder problems or interstitial cystitis should think twice before taking progesterone. Consult with your gynecologist and ask for help in working around all your health problems when choosing any hormone replacement therapy.

In general, any therapeutic decision you make should be agreed upon by you and your doctor. You assess the risks and then work with your physician to minimize them through a health management program. Your preferences count. You may have to shop around to find a doctor who will join you as a partner in your health care, as opposed to the type of physician who says, "Do as I tell you and don't ask why." But the search is worthwhile, and the doctors-as-partners are out there if you look.

Urethral Dilations in Menopause Can Be Harmful

Many women develop bladder infections for the first time in menopause. When they go to the urologist they are told they have a stricture that must be dilated. In this procedure, the urologist inserts gradually larger rods into the urethra and stretches, or dilates, it open. The idea is that you have an obstruction in your urethra that has to be broken open. When urine flows freely, the theory goes, your bladder infections will stop.

As discussed in other chapters, urethral dilations are rarely called for. The procedure is generally useless and painful, and in menopausal women, it can create incontinence.

There is, however, a historical basis for why urologists would believe a postmenopausal woman needs urethral dilations. With the loss of estrogen, a small ring of fibrotic tissue can form in the opening of the urethra. A generation ago, when estrogen replacement therapy was not widely available, some older women would develop this band. It probably was not a prevalent cause of bladder infections.

Nowadays I rarely find this fibrotic ring in older women. Estrogen replacement therapy is prevalent and we just don't see it. But the practice of dilating postmenopausal women has endured. A patient recently said that a urologist told her, "My God, woman! You have the urethra of a three-year-old child!" The patient said she certainly was puzzled by this. How come her urethra had found the Fountain of Youth while the rest of her still looked over sixty-five? In my experience, older women are much less likely to buy this story than are younger women. After all, wouldn't you be skeptical upon learning that you've lived fifty years with a child's urethra and never noticed it before?

If you develop bladder infections at this point in life, assess the situation carefully. Your urethra is probably not guilty. More likely at your age are other problems such as osteoporosis or lumbar strain and lower back problems that prevent your bladder from emptying efficiently. As discussed in Chapter One, back trouble is a prime source of bladder trouble.

If you are dilated, you could temporarily find yourself leaking afterward. As we get older, our bladder necks open up a bit, but the external sphincter comes to the rescue and keeps urine from leaking out. A urethral dilation can paralyze the external sphincter and leave you incontinent for a few days. The leakage goes away but your bladder infections could easily continue.

Anna Maria

When Anna Maria went in for her annual gynecologic checkup, she got a terrible fright. Microscopic amounts of blood were found in her urine. At age forty-nine, she was experiencing hot flashes and had planned to discuss that problem with her doctor. Instead, she heard a whole discourse on what it can mean when blood is found in urine. The worst case was cancer.

In not the best of spirits, Anna Maria came to me for a urologic examination. While it is true that blood in urine is one warning sign of cancer, other things can cause this symptom.

I asked her if she ever noticed blood in her underpants.

"Why, yes," she answered. "When I wipe myself, I sometimes see small amounts of blood on the tissue. It hurts to wipe. Sometimes I just dab the outside."

"Do you feel a little burning sensation after you urinate?"

Surprised, she said, "Yes, it does burn. It feels better if I apply a little pressure to the spot that hurts."

"Have you ever seen any blood in your urine?"

Anna Maria was firm. "Absolutely never. And my gynecologist told me the lab test showed very few blood cells. But she said I should have you check me out anyway."

"Do you smoke?"

No, she had never smoked. Nor had she ever worked around known carcinogens that have been associated with bladder cancer.

On the examining table, I took a close look at Anna Maria's urethra. The cause of her problem was immediately evident.

Like the vagina, the urethra has its own protective layer. When children get what is called bubble bath syndrome, the chemicals in the product inactivate this bacteria-resistant layer. Loss of estrogen can also result in degeneration or loss of this layer, leading to what is called a *caruncle*.

A caruncle is a little growth of tissue stemming from an inflammation at the opening of the urethra. Like a little red tongue, it is an outgrowth of irritated tissue.

I had Anna Maria sit up and look at her urethra with the help of a mirror. Although her caruncle was small, she could see it sticking up like a little flame. It was the source of the minute amount of blood in her urine and the light staining in her underwear. It was the source of the burning sensation she felt when she urinated. "The burning is on the outside," she said, "but I never thought to look for anything with a mirror."

A caruncle is a hallmark of estrogen deficiency in women. But what nature takes away, medicine can sometimes give back. Anna Maria put a dab of estrogen cream on her finger and rubbed it into the caruncle. This was like giving her urethra an artificial protective layer. After several weeks of treatment, the caruncle shrank. Sensitive urethral tissue no longer interacted with the environment. Potential causes of inflammation, such as bacteria from the vagina, would not take hold at the opening of the urethra.

Sometimes caruncles grow too large to be treated with estrogen cream. In that case, the tissue around it can be anesthetized locally in the doctor's office. The caruncle is then snipped off.

Blood in urine is a relative finding. In my opinion, if there are twenty to forty red blood cells in a urine sample looked at under the microscope, full diagnostic tests would be wise. But if there are only two to three red blood cells seen in a typical assay, something less serious may be the cause. The loss of estrogen can, for example, thin the walls of the urethra itself. During and after menopause, the urethra is more fragile and subject to having tiny capillaries burst. These are temporary but may lead to a finding of blood in the urine.

One urinalysis should probably not be the criterion for alarm, especially if the patient has never seen blood in her urine. But if the finding is repeatable and in larger concentrations, the possibilities of more serious diseases should be evaluated.

Betty

Betty came to see me with a common complaint of early menopause. She felt the need to urinate frequently. Where before she could drink lots of fluid and wait hours before voiding—"I've always been a real camel," she said—she now found herself wanting to run to the toilet every half hour. She could repress this urge if she just told herself it was a false signal. But if she gave in, only a little urine came out. It began, she said, "to drive me crazy."

On standard tests, Betty's bladder looked great. Her bladder pressure and flow rates were normal. She could indeed move dirt across the sidewalk. Her back was not troubling her and there were no caruncles. She looked normal.

But her problem could be traced back to that loss of estrogen that accompanies menopause. There are estrogen receptors in the trigone, the triangular area in the base of the bladder. The trigone (fully described in Chapter Five) arises from different embryologic tissue than the rest of the bladder and strongly responds to estrogen. The tissue has what are called *receptor sites,* which are like keyholes to molecules of hormone. When an estrogen molecule encounters a receptor, it locks on. The estrogen then helps maintain a protective GAG layer on the trigone.

As your bladder fills, the trigone is shielded from urine by this protective layer. But when the bladder is half full, tiny molecules in urine stimulate sensory nerves in the trigone that it is time to void.

But when you lose estrogen, the GAG layer thins and it takes only a small amount of urine to defeat the barrier. The result is urinary frequency, as Betty was experiencing.

"You know," she said, "I wet my bed when I was a kid and I had to go to the bathroom all the time. I felt like this back then." Betty had reverted to what I call the teeny-weeny bladder club.

Many women with urinary frequency have insufficient protective lining in their trigones. This can be caused by different factors but the result is almost always frequency.

The solution to Betty's problem was straightforward. When she went on oral estrogen replacement therapy, her symptoms disappeared. The estrogen induced her protective GAG layer to thicken and restore normal bladder function. As Merlys did, she decided to avoid progesterone because it destroys what estrogen builds back up in the bladder.

Many women past menopause also have a problem with their thyroid hormone. I believe this is an issue that is not carefully evaluated by many gynecologists. Thyroid hormone is important for cellular maturation and may be linked, in a complicated interaction, with estrogen and other sex hormones. It exerts very real effects on bladder tissue. I find many patients' symptoms of urinary frequency disappear when they take medication to put their thyroids back into normal range.

Dena

Loss of estrogen can lead to bladder infections along circuitous pathways. One of my favorite examples of this involves Dena. She was a tornado of a woman who bore and raised thirteen children. Dena never sat still. She talked fast. And, as you might expect, she voided fast.

By her own account, Dena sat on the toilet as little as possible. After urinating, she'd dash to her feet and be off to do something more important.

But then Dena developed what some physicians call menopausal cystitis. She had never had a problem with her urinary tract in her life. Then, boom! menopause changed all that.

Actually, Dena had had symptoms of bladder trouble all her life. But she could usually stave off infections by forcing herself to drink quarts of liquids and urinating often. She only used antibiotics when desperate. Moreover, Dena voided with a hard, fast stream thanks to her powerful abdominal muscles. She had used these muscles all her life to help her urinate. And like most women who bear several (even thirteen!) children, Dena had a cystocele, a protrusion or hernia of her bladder wall that held a small amount of urine. Like most cytoceles, Dena's never gave her any trouble, thanks to her strong bladder neck, and she never knew it was there.

Then three things combined to do in Dena's urinary health. First was loss of estrogen, which caused her vagina to lose its tone or elasticity. Then, more than a "weak bladder," she really had a "weak vagina."

Second, as she grew older, the supporting ligaments that held Dena's bladder in position began to lose tone. Both her bladder and her cystocele gradually fell. The cystocele began to sag into her vagina. Her bladder changed shape as its angle of suspension altered.

Third, Dena's bladder never worked right in the first place. She had compression in her lower spine that affected the flow of neurotransmitters to her bladder. But Dena had never had a problem because of her sensational abdominal muscles. These, in effect, made up for her poor bladder function. But when the bladder fell, the abdominal muscles could only push in one direction. They could no longer force her bladder to empty.

Now she was set up for infections. Because she never sat on the toilet long enough to let her cystocele drain, residual urine was left in her bladder. Her bladder did not work properly. Dena got recurrent urinary tract infections.

She responded to bethanechol chloride, a drug that enabled her bladder to contract fully. And she learned to sit on the toilet for an extra thirty seconds or so. If you have a cystocele, you will notice there is a little spurt of urine that comes out after you finish voiding. As the bladder empties, it pulls the cystocele up last, and flattens it. The urine in the cystocele is the last urine out. By squeezing your pelvic floor, you can pull up the bladder muscles and hasten the cystocele to empty.

Dorothy

As we have seen, loss of estrogen affects the vagina, urethra, and bladder. It also affects bone, which is actually an organ of the body.

Dorothy was in her early seventies when she came to see me. She was spry with a jolly outlook on life. But she did have a problem. For seven years, Dorothy had been combatting recurrent urinary tract infections. They came with unsettling regularity. She said she felt as if she were the backbone of the antibiotic industry.

Dorothy's gynecologist held to the school of thought that cystitis is "no big deal," Dorothy explained. "He told me not to worry about it. He said the infections are caused by my thin bladder. Is there such a thing?"

She was worried that bacteria from her bowel could pass through this alleged thin wall and cause her a lot of grief. I assured her that thin bladders are not a cause of cystitis. Her uroflow was abnormal and led clearly to a diagnosis: Her infections could be traced to a lower back problem. "I've always had twinges of discomfort in my back," Dorothy said. "But I ignore it. I'm not a complainer."

Many women suffer silently as Dorothy did. But menopause is a time to speak out about back discomfort. Younger women can experience temporary injury to vertebrae and nerves traveling the spine. Older women can develop osteoporosis, a permanent anatomic change. Between fifteen and twenty million American women have this problem, which tends to accelerate around the time of menopause. It is three times more common in women than in men.

Osteoporosis means "porous bone" and is not a single disease but likely the end result of many disorders. If you think of normal bone to be like Swiss cheese, a bone with osteoporosis has bigger and bigger holes. Such bones grow fragile and eventually collapse. The discs may also degenerate and dry out, compressing nerves in the spine. Osteoporosis is brought on by a chronic gross deficiency of calcium. Because many older people are sedentary, they cut back on total food intake. Unfortunately, they also cut back on vitamins and minerals.

Calcium is an element that is stored in bone. Our bodies use it for a host of basic cellular functions. Whenever the body needs more calcium, it is withdrawn from bone tissue. If for any reason you do not get enough calcium or calcium absorption is impaired or the borrowing goes on too long, the bones lose out. The body keeps withdrawing calcium, which it must have to live, and the bones degenerate.

Everyone begins to lose bone by the age of thirty-five—some say as early as fourteen—but it is gradual. Then at menopause and for about eight years after menopause, bone loss can be very rapid. Some women lose up to 10 percent a year of the bone in the spine. Then the loss resumes its gradual pace.

Osteoporosis is associated with increased fractures of the hip, back, and other bones. White women who undergo premature menopause with hysterectomies and thin women seem to be at highest risk for such fractures. A woman entering menopause has about a 15 percent chance of sustaining a hip fracture in her remaining lifetime. About 40 percent of postmenopausal women who fracture a hip do not return home from the hospital, either dying or remaining in long-term care facilities.

As the holes in bone keep getting bigger, the spaces between the vertebrae (spinal bones) collapse. The vertebrae are pressed against each other. Such changes in the spine affect urinary voiding. Thus menopausal women with urinary problems need to have the health of their backs evaluated.

What happens to the bladder when the vertebrae collapse depends on whether the problem is in the upper back or the lower back. When it happens in the upper back (a condition known as "dowager's hump") (see illustration on page 174), nerves that travel to the bladder are squeezed. The bladder does not get the message to inhibit voiding and the bladder contracts on its own. The primary symptoms are urinary frequency and urgency. As noted earlier, frequency can be brought on through changes in estrogen receptors to the trigone. But osteoporosis of the upper back is another cause.

The lower back presents a different story. When vertebral discs lower down are compressed, the bladder can be completely knocked out of action. Nerves are squeezed and the bladder does not get the message to contract. Urine stays overlong in the bladder and, like a stagnant pool, invites organisms to thrive. The primary symptom is chronic urinary tract infection. Overflow incontinence can also develop.

With osteoporosis these changes are permanent. No amount of exercise or yoga classes will rectify the problem and estrogen therapy will not replace bone mass. But Dorothy was greatly helped by bethanechol chloride, which helped her bladder contract, and the infections cleared up. She also took calcium supplements and learned to eat foods high in calcium, such as leafy dark green vegetables, yogurt, and cheese.

Degenerative arthritis and cracked vertebrae (spondylolisthesis) can also lead to recurrent urinary tract infections. Another woman in her seventies, Hattie, told me proudly that she could hold urine longer than any of her friends. But she developed cystitis precisely because her bladder was not emptying com-

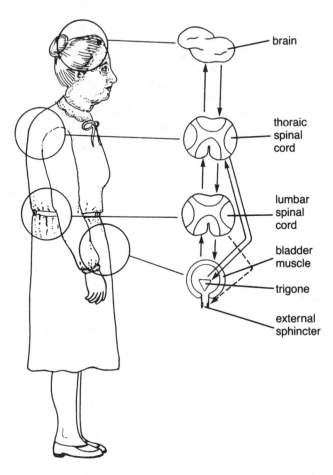

Figure 7-1, Areas of the Body Which Can Cause Urinary Problems

pletely. Her uroflow showed abdominal straining and her cysto-metrogram showed poor voiding pressures. Her problem was traced to degenerative arthritis of the lower spine, a common site of arthritis.

Ruth

The bladder is one of the most sensitive indicators of neuro-logic health. In postmenopausal women, it can forewarn of strokes and other damage to the brain and nervous system.

Ruth was the first person who demonstrated this to me. She was in her seventies and healthy when all of a sudden she became incontinent. She would feel a cramping sensation and urinate uncontrollably. Oddly, whenever she put her hand in cold water, she urinated. This was very inconvenient for washing dishes and doing other household chores.

Ruth's internist, however, could find nothing wrong. Her blood pressure was a little high but not worrisome. The urologic workup in my office, however, showed that her bladder was experiencing uninhibited contractions. It was "firing" all on its own. She urinated when she put her hand in cold water because she was stimulating a well-known but not at all understood feedback mechanism in her nervous system. Nothing was wrong with her back and it was hard to know how to help her. Two months later she had a major stroke.

Ruth was proof that the bladder is one of the most sensitive indicators of neurologic problems. Before her stroke, numerous brain cells had begun to be cut off from oxygen and ceased to function. Some of these nerve cells were involved with her bladder function. As the cells died slowly, her bladder was gradually affected. Finally, the stroke became acute and Ruth went into urinary retention. That is, her bladder ceased working entirely.

Fortunately, Ruth recovered. She went through a physical therapy program and regained control over her bladder.

Since Ruth came to me I have seen several patients, both male and female, with similar symptoms. They are older and previously healthy with bladders that overreact for no discernible reason. Within a few months, they have strokes. I am now convinced that this pattern of urologic findings can predict strokes in some individuals.

In such cases, patients might want to take aspirin every day. This helps prevent blood platelets from clumping together and may ward off a stroke. If you believe you may be at risk, you should discuss with your physician current thoughts on stroke management and prevention.

Ella

Ella was another patient who really stumped me for a time. She was fifty-two, had just gone through menopause, and was not taking estrogen replacement therapy. Although she had had uterine cancer and underwent a hysterectomy, she looked fabulous. "Except for these bladder infections," she said, "I feel better than I ever have."

Ella had no history of bladder infections before menopause. Her uroflow and cystometrogram were normal. Her bladder generated adequate pressures. She had no problems with her back and her urethra looked fine.

Why did she get infections? The only clue was that the infections were related to intercourse. They happened after she and her husband made love.

Ella reaffirmed for me the value of being a woman physician. I have found that women are comfortable confiding in other women. After much discussion, Ella said she was worried about not having enough lubricant in her vagina. "I know women my age dry out and I don't want that to happen. I read in a woman's magazine that one way to avoid infection is to be well lubricatred," she said. Ella then described the lubricant she put on her husband's penis before lovemaking. Ella was following that uncommendable concept, "If a little is good, a lot is better." She frosted his penis with the goo.

The jelly was indirectly responsible for her infections. During intercourse, bacteria adhered to the lubricant which then would be deposited in her urethra. As it stuck to her tissues, bacteria had a chance to collect, grow, and travel to her bladder.

To eliminate infections, Ella learned to use the lubricant appropriately. She put a dab at the vagina's posterior forchette (see Figure 1–7, p. 36) where it would do the most good. This curve at the bottom of the vagina is where most trauma occurs. Here the vagina is vulnerable to tears if the angle of penetration is too high. But if the forchette is lubricated, the vagina is protected.

A word here, too, about sexual positions during menopause. At this time, your urethra is more vulnerable than ever to improper technique. The urethra lacks protective layers and can be traumatized by high angles of penetration. It is not as resilient as when you were younger.

Fortunately, there are many positions other than the missionary approach (male on top) that will not hurt your urethra. When the man enters from the side, the angle of penetration is ideally aligned to the vaginal opening. You can sit on top of him or have him enter from behind as you rest on your hands and knees. Anything that keeps the angle of penetration from stressing your vagina and urethra is fine.

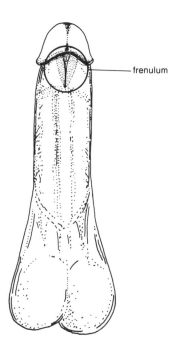

Figure 7-2, The Main Sensory Area of the Penis

It may help you to know how a man is stimulated, so that you can experiment with his anatomy and yours. The main sensory area on his penis is the *frenulum,* a little skin bridge between the head of the penis and the shaft below (see illustration on page 177). It is this part of his penis that needs to be stimulated for him to achieve orgasm. The shaft of his penis is not his erogenous zone. The frenulum can be stimulated without a lot of up and down pumping action. Moreover, the penis does not have to be fully inserted and thrusted for him to feel pleasure. If you hold his penis just part way in your vagina with your pelvic floor muscles, even a slight rocking motion will feel good to you both.

Florence

While loss of estrogen is a major factor in the urinary troubles encountered in menopause, it is not the only problem. The incidence of incontinence rises with age. It is fair to say that women after menopause are leakier than women before menopause. Of course menopause does not *cause* incontinence. But the factors that lead to incontinence are more prevalent the older we get. (See Chapter Six for a detailed discussion of urinary incontinence.)

Around menopause, the overlap of gynecologic and urologic problems seems to increase. My advice is to choose your specialists carefully. Just as you would not want a urologist to deliver your baby or insert an IUD, you may not want a gynecologist to treat your urinary problem with gynecologic procedures.

Florence's story illustrates this point well. She is a fifty-five-year-old grandmother who took up jogging shortly before her fiftieth birthday. "I finally succumbed," she said. "My husband is a runner and now I'm as addicted as he is. I may be slow but I'm steady. I probably do ten to fifteen miles a week and I love it."

Florence is not alone. My office looks out on a road in west Los Angeles that is famous for its jogging path. Hundreds of runners go by all day long. Many, I notice, are women Florence's age.

Two years ago Florence noticed that she was leaking urine while running. The problem had been there to a minor degree before, but now it was worse. She had what is termed mild urinary stress incontinence, a strictly physiologic problem involving loss of support to the bladder neck.

Without thinking much was wrong, Florence went to her gynecologist. She knew women her age tended to leak. She wanted to
know if it could be stopped. She certainly did not intend to give
up running.

The gynecologist examined her and said, "So you leak urine?"

"Yes," said Florence. "But only when running."

"Well," the doctor said, "the reason is that you have a fibroid
[a benign growth] on your uterus. The uterus is pressing down on
your bladder, creating the problem. Your bladder can't fill properly against the mass."

"How big is it?" asked Florence.

"Well, it's about the size of a tennis ball."

Florence thought back to the times she was pregnant. A fetus
gets a lot bigger than a tennis ball and doesn't cause this problem.
She did not have any cramps or bleeding from the fibroid. Why
should it cause trouble?

"This fibroid is taking up space," the gynecologist said. "Your
bladder is too weak to push against it. You're no spring chicken.
It's this constant pressure from the fibroid that's making you leak
urine when you run."

Florence did not like hearing this. Then the doctor said, "The
best solution is a hysterectomy. You're past the age when you're
going to have kids. I guarantee with your uterus out, you won't
leak. It's the best course if you plan to keep running. Otherwise,
you'll get more leaky." The doctor then added, with a wink,
"After I take out your uterus, I'll tighten up your vagina. Your
husband will like that."

Florence was now very worried. Her uterus, despite the fibroid, was healthy. It did not bother her. Did she really need a
hysterectomy? Did she need to be tightened up?

It is highly unusual today that I see a woman in her sixties who
still owns all her parts. There has been a predilection in recent
years for removing uteruses on the following grounds: Why keep
it if you're not going to have any more children? What's the
difference? (Of course, the corollary to this operation in men is
highly frowned upon. They do not undertake such drastic steps
when they decide to have no more children.)

Having your uterus removed *does* make a difference. For some
women, it creates major medical problems. The uterus and bladder are closely aligned; they share supporting ligaments. The

uterus is meant to "press" on the bladder and, as the British urologist Mr. Turner-Warwick says, when the uterus is taken away, the bladder misses it. Any time the uterus enlarges, it does so without altering bladder function. This is an important point to remember.

Just as the urethra is often incorrectly blamed for bladder problems, so the uterus is often blamed for a bladder problem.

There is a widely held myth concerning postmenopausal women and fibroids of the uterus. Uterine fibroids, as Florence's doctor said, enlarge the uterus and thereby press on the bladder. He believes that this causes symptoms of frequency because the bladder is unable to fill properly, or that it causes the bladder to leak. This theory is not correct. The biggest "fibroid" of all is a nine-pound fetus. Such enlargement of the uterus is perfectly normal and does not alter bladder capacity. As will be discussed in Chapter Eight, you may urinate more frequently when pregnant because you are "voiding for two," but the size of your bladder does not change. It does not make sense that a fibroid would have a different impact on the bladder than pregnancy does. Both enlarge the uterus. And like pregnancy, fibroids have no bearing on bladder function. Hysterectomies have never made a bladder function better.

Why does this belief—that the uterus is to blame for a leaky bladder—persist in gynecology? There is a probable answer. In the extreme condition of uterine prolapse, the uterus falls and pulls the bladder down with it. The bladder neck is opened and women leak urine. The most effective treatment really is to remove the uterus. But I believe that many gynecologists have applied this principle to uteruses and bladders that are in proper position. The extreme case has been generalized for all cases.

At the same time, many gynecologists were taught that urinary frequency during pregnancy is a function of the uterus pressing on the bladder. As will be discussed in Chapter Eight, this is really not the case until the very latter stage of pregnancy; women urinate frequently in pregnancy for other reasons.

Gynecologists view the bladder from the perspective of the uterus and tend to overlook the urologic explanations for incontinence. It is only as more gynecologists become interested in the bladder (which seems to be happening) that these "gynocentric," to coin a word, explanations will become less common.

Florence's problem was with her bladder neck. If you recall, we stay dry when the pressure in the urethra is greater than the pressure in the bladder. When support ligaments to the bladder neck lose tone, the bladder neck starts to pull open. Then only the external sphincter in the urethra keeps us dry and a sudden "stress" such as coughing, laughing, sneezing or the pounding motion of jogging can be enough to let urine past the sphincter. Then we leak.

Fortunately, Florence came to me for a second opinion. She had never had surgery in her life and was not anxious to undergo the scalpel. In her workup, we discovered she did not have a csytocele and that her whole problem lay with her bladder neck. She was an ideal candidate for Teflon injection into the bladder neck, an office procedure using a local anesthetic, fully described in Chapter Six. After the procedure, Florence kept running, and in fact sometimes waves as she passes by my office.

Alice

When Alice was forty-seven, she began to have trouble urinating. Her gynecologist said her uterus was enlarged and it had best come out. "He did find tumors and I am convinced it was a necessary operation," she said. But six weeks after surgery, she developed intense bladder pain. It was a relentless, burning pressure that left Alice devastated.

The ancient Greeks thought there was a connection between a woman's emotions and her genitals. The Greek word for uterus is *hystera* and thus we call the surgical removal of the organ a *hysterectomy*. Hysterectomies are the most frequently performed major operations in the United States. In 1984 alone, 700,000 hysterectomies were performed in the United States.

Some physicians routinely take out the ovaries at the same time they remove the uterus. The attitude is that once you've had children, the uterus and the ovaries become useless, bleeding, symptom-producing, and potentially cancer-bearing organs. But there is now clear evidence that the ovaries are important throughout your life, even in old age. They should not be removed unless they are diseased. If they are taken out, you will experience what amounts to man-made menopause.

There is confusion over the terms used for this operation. Most people think of a "total hysterectomy" as removal of the uterus, fallopian tubes, and ovaries. In medical terminology the removal of both fallopian tubes and ovaries along with the uterus is a "total hysterectomy and bilateral salpingo-oophorectomy." When the uterus and cervix are removed it is properly called a "total hysterectomy." In a "subtotal hysterectomy," the cervix is left in.

The uterus can be taken out in two ways, through the vagina or through an incision in the abdomen. The vaginal procedure is indicated when the uterus is small enough and pelvic ligaments large enough to allow easy access through the vagina.

If you refer to Figure 5-3, The Complete Female Urinary System, page 132, you will notice that the ureters (the tubes that carry urine from the kidneys) cross the ovaries on their way down to the bladder. One well-known complication of a hysterectomy is accidental cutting of the ureters. This is usually recognized immediately and repaired, but if it is not, fever and pain occur on the injured side right after surgery. If still not recognized, within one or two days the symptoms of a kidney infection can arise.

Another complication is not so well known. It involves the network of nerves discussed in Chapter Two that carries chemicals first identified in the brain—the neurotransmitters serotonin, norepinephrine, and acetylcholine. These nerves run from the brain, to the heart, to the gut, to the bladder, and to the clitoris. Target tissue along the pathway contains receptor sites, the exact locations where the neurotransmitters bind. The pathway of nerves is highly coordinated by the brain and controls the body's fight or flight response. Signals are sent to stimulate or prevent transmission of these substances.

Although the total pathway of these nerves is not yet identified, there is good evidence that they traverse the ovaries, cross the ureters, and enter the bladder from behind. From there they travel between the bladder and vagina. As pointed out, on one side, nerves go to the trigone. Just opposite, they go to the erogenous G spot in the vagina. The nerves then continue to the urethra and on out to the clitoris.

Many women complain they lose vaginal sensitivity after a hysterectomy. Some have problems achieving orgasm. If we assume this set of nerves exists in women, perhaps we have an explanation for such loss. Is it not possible that, for some women, these nerves are cut accidentally during hysterectomies? Might this explain their symptoms?

Interestingly, these nerves have been found and fully traced in men. When the nerves are cut accidentally during a prostate operation, men become impotent. Thus urologists have learned how to avoid damaging the nerves of men. But urologists have had little interest in proving the existence of these nerves in women and learning how not to damage them.

Of course, not every woman who has her ovaries and uterus removed will suffer damage to these nerves. Many are lucky. But, as my office charts attest, the problem is far from rare.

Marilyn

Within days after her hysterectomy, Marilyn experienced intense burning in the lower part of her bladder. We knew it was too soon for loss of estrogen to create this symptom. And she felt no frequency and had no infections; the problem was burn.

She had developed one variation of the disease that we call interstitial cystitis. There were other contributing factors to Marilyn's problem but the main precipitating event was her hysterectomy. It is possible that the nerves conducting the fight or flight neurotransmitters to her bladder had been severed. This would alter the balance of those transmitters in her bladder. Certainly one of them, serotonin, has been implicated with burn to tissue.

Within a few months, Marilyn began to notice that certain foods made the burn more intense. Wine, cheese, and chocolate were at the top of the list. These foods contain substances that are converted into serotonin by the body.

Working on the assumption that a nerve feedback mechanism might be out of sync, I prescribed a medication that blocks the action of serotonin. Marilyn went on a diet low in serotonin-promoting foods. Her burn improved markedly. (See Chapter Eleven for more good news about how diet can help.)

This entire mechanism, however, is not well understood and Marilyn is not free of all discomfort. It is an area of active research at the Interstitial Cystitis Foundation. With Marilyn's continued and cheerful help, we hope to find the answers.

In the meantime, gynecologists are pioneering new methods

that should make hysterectomies less prevalent. For example, uterine bleeding can be treated with lasers that cauterize or seal the bleeding sites; the uterus does not necessarily have to come out. Thus physicians are learning how to heal from within the organ.

Women today are much more assertive about their health care. This is particularly true in menopause, as women take responsibility for their health. It is never too late to do so. With information about how your body changes, you can enter menopause with a very positive mind set. Like Mami Estah, you can plan new beginnings, do the things you never dared or had time for, create a satisfying lifestyle.

Many women who are fifty and over today are excellent role models for younger women. They choose to live full lives that their daughters are proud of and will choose to emulate when they grow up. If you look around, you will see this gift that older women are giving to younger women flourishing everywhere.

Points to remember:

- A hysterectomy is not a cure for bladder problems.
- Estrogen and progesterone therapies have pros and cons.
- Be sure to get enough calcium and eat a proper diet.

EIGHT

Avoiding Cystitis During Pregnancy

When Miriam was six months pregnant, her obstetrician found bacteria in her urine. She had just gone in for her regular checkup and her urinalysis tested positive for E. coli. Her physician telephoned her immediately. The instant that bacteria such as *E. coli,* enterococcus, or proteus are seen in a pregnant woman's urine, an alarm is sounded. It is well known that infected urine is associated with premature labor, and sometimes the fetus does not survive. Therefore, this condition is not to be taken lightly.

It was Miriam's first pregnancy and by every routine measure she was doing extremely well. She looked and felt fine. She had gained the right amount of weight. She continued her work as a city attorney, and other than needing more sleep, her life had not changed much because of her pregnancy.

But now her doctor told her there was true cause for concern. He called her in for another examination but could find nothing wrong. A second urinalysis also tested positive for bacterial infection. Thinking an expert in urinary tract function could shed light on the matter, he referred Miriam to a urologist.

When Miriam came to my office, she was upset. She didn't really want to see another physician but she did want her baby to be healthy. Her "problem," she said, was that she felt fine. She didn't feel as if she were ill.

After I asked some questions, Miriam finally blurted out, "But I feel perfectly well! You'd think that if I had an infection I'd feel some symptoms. What is it about pregnancy? Does being pregnant somehow take away the symptoms of cystitis?"

Miriam was concerned and I couldn't blame her. Every woman referred to me for asymptomatic cystitis during pregnancy is greatly distressed. It is a confounding problem. You don't want to take a chance of promoting premature labor. But if there are no symptoms, what could be the matter?

I told Miriam to give me another urine sample, cautioning her to make sure she caught the urine in midstream. Then I took a urine sample from her bladder using a catheter. The next day, there was good news: The urine in her bladder was sterile, but the urine she had caught for culturing was contaminated. Therefore, it was only something in the way she had voided that was causing the contamination.

The Shelf Syndrome

Unlike most urologists, I have been pregnant and have delivered a baby. This experience has afforded me a different perspective on questions of urologic health during pregnancy.

When I was about six months pregnant, I began to notice that I had damp underwear most of the time. I was immediately concerned. Was I becoming incontinent? You're not supposed to leak urine when you're pregnant. I wasn't feeling any unusual urges to urinate. In fact, like Miriam, I felt great.

Then one day, as I was sitting on the toilet mulling over the damp underwear problem in my mind, the answer struck me. There I was sitting back on the seat, with my hands folded on my abdomen. I called this my "shelf," that little bridge between your chest wall and the uterus. This shelf allows you to do all sorts of unique things such as balancing books on it or hiding needed surgical instruments from the scrub nurse in the operating room. And it stays with you to the end of your pregnancy.

I realized that I was voiding differently because of my shelf.

When I was not pregnant, I had always leaned forward, spread my legs, and let the urine stream wash off the perineum. But now I was sitting back on the toilet seat because with the extra bulk it was more comfortable that way. I also had my legs together in front of me to offset the imbalance from leaning back.

When I voided in this position, I was allowing urine to flow back up into the vagina. Later, the urine seeped out causing the wet underpants. Such intravaginal reflux of urine, I thought, must be very common in pregnant women. We all get these shelves and we all probably like to lean back when we urinate.

The problem, of course, is that urine draining out of the vagina will easily be contaminated with bacteria. Therefore pregnant women who reflux urine into their vaginas might be misdiagnosed as having bladder infections.

I asked Miriam if she had damp underpants.

"Why, yes I do," she said. "Most of the time. But I thought it was just excess secretions from my vagina with pregnancy and all."

"Do you sit back when you void?"

"Yes I do," she said. "I have trouble leaning forward because I'm too big." And thus, using a common sense approach, we solved her mystery. Once she understood what she was doing, she learned to lean forward by spreading her legs wide apart to make room for her enlarged uterus. The damp underwear stopped and her urine samples in the future were sterile.

I believe that genuine bladder infections during pregnancy are less common than is thought. Intravaginal reflux of urine, this "shelf syndrome," should be ruled out before antibiotics are prescribed as a result of contaminated urine. The lone finding of bacteria in urine is not satisfactory grounds that you have a bladder infection. The urinalysis is not the only thing to take into consideration.

However, the fact that bacteria-laden urine is constantly present in underwear could lead to bacterial infection of the urethra. When your physician discovers you have infected urine, he or she will sound the alarm and your gynecologist may assume you have a genuine serious bladder infection. He or she may then prescribe suppressive antibiotic therapy to prevent the danger of premature contractions. *But if you don't have a bladder infection, you are taking the drugs unnecessarily.* And, since antibiotics are known to cross the placental barrier, the baby is likewise needlessly exposed to medications.

How to Give a Urine Sample

You should know how to give a urine sample during pregnancy. As part of prenatal care, women routinely give such samples to test for bacteria, glucose, blood, protein, or other factors not present in normal urine.

When you give a sample, be sure that urine does not backflow into your vagina. The best way to go about this is to lean forward and *half stand up* when you void. *Lift your buttocks off the toilet seat and put your weight onto your thighs*. In this position, you can look down and see what you're doing. When you urinate in this half standing position, the stream will drop down and not wash the perineum. You can catch some in the container, knowing it won't contain bacteria from the vagina.

Don't sit down on the toilet seat and place the container underneath hoping that the stream will be caught well enough. Your pelvis is tilted in the wrong direction, causing urine to flow back over the perineum. Attempts at catching this will only result in pubic hair and skin contaminating the container and urine.

It is important whenever you void during pregnancy that you don't give in to the shelf. *Always lean forward and spread your legs apart*. After you void, you might also take a piece of toilet tissue and dab it into the vagina. This catches some of the backflowing urine.

Hopefully, by properly catching a urine sample, you can show that you do not have a urinary tract infection just because bacteria showed up in your urine. If your urine tests positively for bacteria and you feel fine, ask to give another sample for culture. This should be done *as a catheterized sample* and compared to your voided one.

You can also monitor your urine at home throughout pregnancy with home test kits, put out by different manufacturers. With these you can test urine for blood, glucose, bacteria, pH, or proteins.

If you have a history of bladder infections, these tests are useful. If you develop sudden feelings of urinary frequency on a Saturday night (and doesn't it always seem to happen then, when physicians are hard to locate?), you can find out right away if there is cause for concern.

But, I want to emphasize, some things that indicate a urologic problem in a nonpregnant woman may turn out to be normal in a pregnant woman. Not every "abnormal" finding in blood or urine is a sure sign of urologic disease during pregnancy. So before considering what to do if you *do* have a genuine infection of the upper or lower urinary tract during pregnancy, you should understand what normal changes your kidneys, ureters, bladder, and urethra undergo during those remarkable nine months.

Water Retention: When Not to Worry

When you are pregnant, you can develop any urologic problem that might also affect a nonpregnant woman. During pregnancy, however, such problems are compounded by profound physiologic changes in your body plus the presence of a rapidly growing fetus. This combination of factors makes it very difficult to diagnose and treat urologic disorders in pregnant women. Conventional techniques such as X-rays, cystoscopy, and surgery are used only as a last resort. However, in recent years the new technique of ultrasound is shedding light on what the urinary tract really looks like during pregnancy. As with cystitis, the answers are still evolving; not all the information is in.

It is known that during pregnancy your body undergoes some extraordinary changes. Early on, you produce large amounts of the female hormone estrogen. It elevates a substance in blood plasma called *angiotensin,* which increases the kidneys' filtration rates. Thus early on blood flow to the kidneys increases so that you can filter more toxins, including those produced by the fetus. This is natural and necessary, and such increased blood flow is maintained at fairly constant levels all through your pregnancy.

Moreover, when you are pregnant, you retain fluids. This is because your kidneys become very adept at reclaiming any sodium, or salt, that passes through them; not much is lost to urine. As a result, some *edema,* or "water retention," is normal during pregnancy.

How can you tell if you have edema? Look for the thinnest part of your leg along the shinbone. Press in with your finger, count to three, and release. The degree of impression left by your finger indicates how much edema you have. You have some excess fluid on board if there is a mild depression. If you made a deep cavity, you have excessive fluid retention and should see a physician.

Some women find the edema of pregnancy an upsetting side effect but you should be aware that there is a reason behind it.

First consider what happens when you are not pregnant. Your kidneys must continuously filter blood at a proper, controlled rate. When for various reasons (changes in posture, salt intake, drugs, or other factors) blood pressure falls, so that the blood flow through the kidneys falls below the normal range, your kidneys are stimulated to excrete an enzyme called *renin*. This in turn stimulates your body's smallest blood vessels to constrict, reducing volume of the circulatory system and increasing blood pressure. It also stimulates the adrenal glands to secrete a hormone that promotes reabsorption of salt and water by the kidneys. More fluid stays in the circulatory system and this also elevates blood pressure. The higher blood pressure signals the kidneys to no longer release renin. The whole system operates on a feedback mechanism.

In pregnancy, the same mechanism is present but in much higher levels. You are now filtering the blood of two people. Since the kidneys of the fetus are not yet working, your kidneys serve as the filtration system for both of you.

The increased edema that is so often seen with pregnancy should, in the absence of chronic high blood pressure, be viewed as just a normal physiologic response to pregnancy. You should not have to limit your salt or take diuretics unless the edema is excessive.

Some pregnant women strive to maintain their slim body image by taking diuretic medication during pregnancy, often without the knowledge or approval of their obstetrician. My advice is, don't do it. Edema is a normal response to pregnancy. The state is temporary and you should not interfere with the natural course of pregnancy for reasons of vanity.

Glucose or Protein in Urine During Pregnancy: When Not to Worry

It used to be thought that finding glucose in urine was a sign of latent diabetes; if glucose showed up in your urine during pregnancy, the doctor might suspect you are diabetic. Recent work, however, has shown this not to be true.

Remember the kidneys are working overtime during pregnancy. They are filtering what your system makes as well as what the fetus makes. At times your filtering mechanism can be overwhelmed by this double load. When that happens, excess substances can be dumped into urine.

For example, the clearing mechanism can be overwhelmed by a temporarily high load of sugar. Excess sugar is simply dumped out into urine, even though blood levels of sugar, or glucose, are normal. So if you are told you have sugar in your urine during pregnancy, don't panic. This does not automatically mean you are diabetic. Ask for a glucose tolerance test to see if your blood sugar levels are remaining in the normal range.

In a similar manner, protein is sometimes found in the urine of pregnant women. This may be due to the same mechanism of the protein load outstripping the ability of the kidneys to reabsorb all of it.

To repeat: Finding glucose or protein in urine is not an absolute diagnosis that you have a metabolic problem. It can be a normal occurrence during pregnancy.

However, if you are a diabetic and you are pregnant, take very special care to maintain proper glucose metabolism. In the past, women with kidney diseases in general were told to never get pregnant because they would be unable to handle the complex physiologic changes of pregnancy and childbirth. Today, with drugs to control edema and high blood pressure, as well as more aggressive management of pregnancy, many more women are completing pregnancies despite abnormal kidney function.

However, in this situation it is important to find a gynecologist and nephrologist who can deal with high-risk obstetric problems. Before you get pregnant, discuss with them the types of things that may be necessary and what the risks are to your general health.

Reducing Your Risk of Kidney Stones During Pregnancy

Some women develop kidney stones during pregnancy. This may be related to their high intake of calcium. Some women eat calcium like crazy in their zeal to "give my baby strong bones," but excess calcium in your diet in the absence of extra magnesium can lead to kidney stones.

It happens like this. When you eat certain foods, such as some green leafy vegetables, you increase the amount of the substance *oxalate* in your bloodstream. Oxalate is derived from an acid found in certain plants. It is generally excreted in urine as an unwanted, toxic substance. Oxalate carries a negative charge, and as it passes through the kidneys, it tends to bind electrically to elements that carry a positive charge. Calcium and magnesium are such positively charged elements. They attach to oxalate in the urine.

As it happens, calcium is not very soluble in water. When it binds with oxalate, it has the tendency to form crystals. These can grow into what are known as calcium-oxalate kidney stones. Magnesium, however, is more soluble in water. When it binds with oxalate, it tends to carry the substance out of the kidney in urine. It binds to oxalate before calcium has a chance to do so and serves as a protecting agent against stones.

You can see how you might get into trouble by taking in a lot of calcium by eating green leafy vegetables (which are good for you) and not adding magnesium to help rid your kidneys of oxalate.

Many prenatal vitamins contain calcium and magnesium. Others do not. Check your prescription and talk it over with your physician. For best urologic health, both elements should be taken. Another supplement using calcium citrate also inhibits calcium-oxalate crystallization. It contains a component of citrus fruits.

Recent studies conducted in England stress the importance of taking prenatal vitamins in other ways. They found there is an association between not taking vitamins (especially early in pregnancy) and neural tube defects in infants. Such defects involve malformation of the spinal cord and brain. Since neural tube defects occur in about one in every 1,000 births, doctors who did the study recommend strongly that women take vitamins even when they are trying to get pregnant.

It is extremely important that you keep yourself hydrated during pregnancy. Some women, in trying to maintain a slim figure, will dehydrate themselves. They forget pregnancy is temporary and not a time for great vanity. This puts them at risk for stones and risks the baby's well-being. Remember, your urinary tract is designed to clear wastes from the fetus as well as from your body. I do not adhere to the drink-eight-glasses-of-water-a-day school but think you should use common sense. Adjust your water intake according to climate and activity. If your urine is so concentrated that you can't read a newspaper through it, you need more fluids.

The rate of incidence of kidney stones in pregnant and nonpregnant women of the same age is really no different. The most common signs of stone disease in pregnancy include pain in the groin and back, with tenderness, fever, nausea and vomiting, blood and pus in the urine, and even frequency or irritation while urinating. However, stones can also be present without any noticeable symptoms. A woman who has had more than one child seems to be more prone to kidney stones than the woman having her first child. This may be because earlier pregnancies alter the urinary tract, allowing changes to the protective layer of the kidneys to occur more readily.

As you can imagine, kidney stones during pregnancy present a problem. An abbreviated X-ray can be done to evaluate quickly whether or not a stone is present. Ultrasound may be tried but tends to present a confusing image; it is hard to tell if the swelling of the kidney is caused by the obstruction of a stone or just by the normal changes found in pregnancy.

Several less insoluble substances in urine can abnormally crystallize into kidney stones. Calcium phosphate stones tend to grow quickly. Calcium oxalate stones are slow growing and tend to have sharp jagged edges. Uric acid stones are seen in people with a family history of gout. Exactly what causes these different stones is not known. Nevertheless, these stones can be dissolved by alkalizing urine with sodium bicarbonate tablets and a low uric acid diet. When the pH factor of urine is kept above 8, uric acid stones tend to dissolve away.

Magnesium phosphate stones are a different variety. They cannot be dissolved by altering urinary pH. These stones, which cannot be picked up by a single X-ray (called a flat plate) but require other imaging techniques, often get infected (another name for them, in fact, is "infected stones"). Infected stones tend to occur in women who have chronic kidney infections and rarely occur in those without that medical history. They are treated with antibiotics.

Any stone can become lodged in the renal pelvis or in a ureter. When this happens, urine is prevented from flowing into the bladder, and pain and infection can ensue.

Ovarian vein syndrome, which is discussed below, may also be involved with some kidney stone formation during pregnancy. In this syndrome, the right ureter becomes partially blocked. As a result calyxes, the cuplike structures that drain urine from above, become distended by the increasing pressure of urine. As in bladder tissue, this distension, or stretching, alters the protective GAG layer of the calyxes.

Instead of an electrically neutral surface, an electrically charged surface is now exposed. Charged elements in urine are magnetically attracted to damaged surface tissue. Also, urine drainage is not as fast or efficient when a ureter is partially blocked. The renal pelvis therefore turns into a kind of reservoir. Stones may then form. Like the sugar crystals you grow in water, stone crystals begin to aggregate in stagnant urine. Kidney stones are more frequently found late in pregnancy as the ureteral obstruction increases.

In my experience, however, most kidney stones that arise during pregnancy tend to pass about six weeks after delivery. Most women never know they have them until their bodies return to a normal "hydrodynamic" state. That is, once their hormones resume a nonpregnant balance and the ureters become less dilated, the stone dislodges and passes on its own accord.

Postpartum stone disease may be prevented by taking care to eat a balanced diet with special attention to the proper balance of minerals and vitamins and maintaining adequate fluid intake.

Why Your Ureters Will Dilate in Pregnancy

It has been known for over 100 years that one region of the urinary tract dilates significantly in about 90 percent of all pregnant women: where the ureters, the tubes that carry urine down to your bladder, meet the kidney. This whole upper portion of the urinary tract, called the *renal pelvis,* enlarges when you are pregnant. This is seen to occur as early as the sixth to the tenth week of pregnancy and reaches its peak around twenty-two to twenty-four weeks. It is a normal physiologic change that causes no problem unless there is some complication, such as a urinary tract infection.

Urologists have given this phenomenon some thought and are still coming up with reasons to explain why it occurs. Today there are three main theories. All may be correct.

The first is based on principles of what happens when you obstruct the flow of water. When you step on a garden hose, less water comes through the line. Pressure builds behind the point where you put your foot. Similarly, as your uterus enlarges, it partially obstructs and puts pressure on the ureter. The increased urinary flow coming down the ureter has less of a caliber to get through. Therefore, the ureter expands in response to the partial obstruction.

However, dilation of the upper part of the urinary tract occurs very early in pregnancy, before the uterus is big enough to put pressure on the ureter. Thus a second theory has been proposed. Early in pregnancy, hormones act on smooth muscle in the uterus, permitting it to expand to hold the growing fetus. The nearby ureters are also composed of smooth muscle, which propels urine toward the bladder. And there is a smooth muscle lining in the bladder. Thus hormones that expand the smooth muscle of the uterus probably affect smooth muscles in the urinary tract. The ureters and the bladder enlarge.

Finally, it is theorized that ureters expand because more fluid is draining through the system. You are simply clearing more urine. And, like the system of the diabetic with increased urine flow, your system expands to cope with the volume.

Interestingly, this dilation of the upper part of the urinary tract is not seen in animals that walk on all fours. It is found only in primates and is thought to be a consequence of our upright posture. Because of gravity, the abdominal contents of four-legged animals fall forward, away from the ureters.

Most pregnant women experience some degree of ureteral obstruction throughout most of the day. This is why lying down and putting your feet up feels so good. You are reducing congestion in the veins around your uterus and urinary tract. And you relieve some of that pressure on your lower back. At the same time, this change in position increases the amount of blood flowing through the kidney. Your system is relieved overall.

If you lie on the opposite side from the side that hurts, you may be able to relieve pressure by causing the contents of your abdomen to fall away from the area being obstructed. Our mothers and grandmothers knew this instinctively but now there is a medical explanation for why it helps. The swelling of kidneys during pregnancy often can be managed simply by changing positions. You should sleep and rest on your side.

There is a related condition of pregnancy that you may hear mentioned if you experience a backache in your right side as pregnancy progresses. It is fairly common and usually no cause for concern. It is called *ovarian vein syndrome*. To see what happens, see the illustration on page 197. A system of veins stems from both the right and left ovaries. The veins from the left ovary enter into the main renal vein. But veins from the right ovary join and drain into the vena cava. This causes the vein to cross over the right ureter. When you are not pregnant, this body architecture has no untoward consequences.

But when you are pregnant, a problem can arise. First, as discussed, the ureters expand. At the same time, the veins expand as they clear more blood from the uterine complex. If the enlarged vein compresses the right ureter, obstruction can ensue. The system gets clogged and you feel pain in your right upper back.

Most of the time this condition is just a nuisance. But sometimes the obstruction becomes so great that a true kidney infection, complete with fever and chills, follows. Then you and your doctor are faced with a real dilemma. The condition itself is self-limiting. Once pregnancy is over, the vein returns to normal size and the ureter functions normally. Women with kidney infection resulting from ovarian vein syndrome may be given antibiotics to save their kidney from damaging bacteria and to prevent premature labor. Once the baby is delivered, however, an IVP is necessary to ensure that no anatomic problem exists that would continue to affect the kidneys.

Some women have an abnormal urinary tract that works fine until they become pregnant. The physiologic changes that ensue serve to unmask a latent kidney or bladder problem. It is not until their systems have to work for two that, say, a mild reflux problem is manifested. If you ever develop a fever during pregnancy along with back pain, urinary frequency, and burning when you urinate, you should seek immediate medical attention. If you

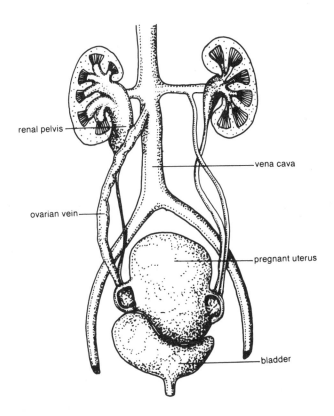

Figure 8-1, Ovarian Vein Compressing the Ureter

have pyelonephritis (an infection of the kidney), the usual treatment is antibiotic therapy targeted to the organism that is cultured from urine. If you have this problem, your doctor will want to follow your pregnancy very closely.

Bladder Changes During Pregnancy

Your bladder, too, undergoes normal physiologic changes in response to pregnancy.

One of the earliest changes is in response to hormone changes. Your trigone, the sensory area of the bladder that signals you have to void, contains numerous receptors for the hormones estrogen and progesterone. Molecules of these hormones affect the trigone, binding or attaching to receptor sites, just as keys fit into locks.

In early pregnancy the body rapidly increases the release of estrogen and progesterone. These hormones, in turn, overstimulate the trigone. Until the bladder becomes accustomed to the higher levels, the trigone responds by making you want to void frequently. This happens around the sixth week after conception and is an early indication that you are indeed pregnant. In those early weeks, many women report they have to void often at night, even though the fetus is too small as yet to be producing much extra waste.

Increased hormone levels also serve to increase the elasticity of smooth muscle within your bladder, allowing you to carry and hold more urine than usual. It must accommodate the increased filtration load of your kidneys, which are now working overtime.

You may in fact notice that you void more often in pregnancy. This is because you are voiding for two. You are probably drinking more fluids as well, to meet the needs of two bodies. Although the uterus is enlarging, it does not—contrary to popular belief—press down on the bladder, so that it has less room and needs to be emptied more often.

As you can see from the illustrations here, the bladder may assume all sorts of shapes and positions during pregnancy. It sits in front of the uterus and it flattens out somewhat as the fetus grows. While the uterus may even push out the inside of your belly button, the bladder only changes shape. It does *not* lose capacity.

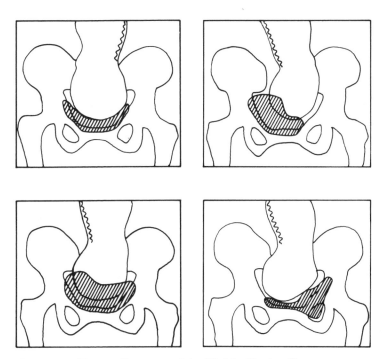

Figure 8-2, Various Positions of the Bladder During Pregnancy

Only in the last month or so of pregnancy does the greatly enlarged womb have the effect of truly crowding the bladder. The bladder could still handle a high volume of urine but it just doesn't have the room. You may develop urinary frequency around this time, since there is no space left in your pelvic area for the baby and a full bladder at the same time.

Safely Treating Bladder Infections in Pregnancy

When Nancy came to see me, she was seven and a half months pregnant and frightened. Her gynecologist had found bacteria in her urine. He told her the dangers of cystitis during pregnancy and she was, of course, deeply concerned.

Unlike Miriam, Nancy had symptoms other than a positive urine culture. She felt burning and pain when she voided. Her urine was a smoky color and it contained blood. She had frequency and felt pressure.

Nancy had been given ampicillin to knock out the infection. Penicillin and some of its variations have been used for decades now in treating bladder infections during pregnancy with no obvious ill effects in the majority of people. Nevertheless, these drugs are used cautiously and only when indicated, for no drugs are 100 percent safe during pregnancy.

But Nancy was concerned that if she had to take an antibiotic during pregnancy she might need to do the same after she delivered. She came to me to find out why she had an infection in the first place and how she might avoid having it happen again after pregnancy.

Nancy said she had never had a bladder infection before in her life, and it came as a real shock to her. "If I'd had these all the time, like my friend Carole does," she said, "I might be less upset."

My first step was to give her a uroflow exam. Since Nancy was pregnant, we could eliminate mechanical obstruction caused by the diaphragm.

Just as I suspected, Nancy's uroflow showed primary bladder dysfunction. Her urine stream was weak and intermittent. It was certainly not strong enough to move dirt on a sidewalk. The nerves stemming from her lower back to her bladder were not fully working. Nancy's bladder could not generate a good contraction. Leftover urine stagnated in her bladder. Eventually, she got an infection.

Upon questioning, Nancy said she never had an out-and-out back problem, nothing that ever landed her in bed. But it did hurt at times when she was overzealous in gardening or in lifting heavy objects. But, she said, "My back has really been bothering me in the last few months. The extra weight of the baby is a real strain."

Often pregnancy will tip the scales of an incipient lower back problem. You may stand differently, swaying your back, to accommodate your belly. This lordosis puts strain on the back, particularly if you wear high heels.

If lower back strain leads to cystitis when you are not pregnant, bethanechol chloride helps to correct the problem while strengthening your back and correcting your posture. Unfortunately, this drug should not be taken in pregnancy. It can cause uterine contractions and therefore lead to miscarriage or premature delivery.

Nancy began special back exercises, recommended by her obstetrician, to strengthen her abdominal and lower back muscles. She also wore a maternity girdle to maintain firm back support. She avoided that duck waddle walk favored by pregnant women and straightened up as much as possible.

After she delivered her baby, her lower back problem was resolved. A uroflow now demonstrated a good flow. Nancy was happy. And she also knew that should she ever develop another bladder infection, pregnant or not pregnant, she could likely trace the problem to her lower back.

More often than not, women who develop bladder infections during pregnancy have a previous history of recurrent urinary tract infections. There is something not right in the way their bladders work. Thus, if you have recurrent urinary tract infections, I urge you to have your situation evaluated before you get pregnant. Pregnancy puts an enormous stress on your body and it is prudent to be as healthy as you can before going through it.

Beware of Exercising for Two

During this age of physical fitness, many women are tempted to continue vigorous exercise throughout their pregnancy. It is certainly possible to do so—with some modifications. You don't want to exercise in a way that could injure your lower back and possibly promote bladder infections during pregnancy.

Some exercise books and videotapes—even those designed for pregnant women—contain harmful exercises. Check with your obstetrician before undertaking such a regimen. You might bring the books or tapes to your doctor's office so you can review the steps together.

Use your better judgment before putting yourself in contorted positions. Pregnancy is a time to forget that slim self-image. You cannot deliver your baby and wear your tightest fitting jeans home afterward.

Having been pregnant, I understand the vanity of wanting to maintain your former self-image. In my case, there was a great concern not to show that I was pregnant. I was in residency training. This meant that I was treating patients, and my professors worried that a pregnant female surgeon would disturb some people. But, as I soon learned, it is senseless to try to hide pregnancy. You can only cause harm to yourself and the unborn baby.

Use common sense and take good care of yourself during pregnancy. Your body will return to its former self soon enough.

Solving Postpartum Urologic Problems

The final moment arrives. You've made it through nine months and, at last, that little package you've been waiting for is placed in your arms. You count your blessings. But later on that day, you realize you can't urinate.

Don't panic. This is a fairly common problem. It is temporary. As the baby came through the birth canal, its head pressed against the nerves that go into your bladder and urethra. These nerves may become temporarily paralyzed. There may be some swelling in the tissue. Usually this problem resolves itself in twenty-four hours. It is nothing to worry about.

Pat experienced this problem briefly and was then fine. She went home the day after her baby was born. Everything was going along smoothly until about one month after delivery. She and her husband resumed active intercourse. Then Pat developed her very first bladder infection.

She went to her gynecologist, who reassured Pat that bladder infections are sometimes seen in postpartum women and it is nothing to worry about. Pat took an antibiotic and the infection cleared up—but for only two days. Then she developed a second infection. She took more antibiotics, followed by another infection. At this point, Pat was very concerned. There had been nothing wrong with her before the baby was born. She feared that maybe everything falls apart after childbirth.

Pat came to my office for a urologic workup. She looked healthy. Her uroflow, IVP, and cystometrogram were normal. What could be her problem?

Pat had an infected Skene's gland. Skene's glands are located at the opening of the urethra and secrete wetting agents that help keep tissue healthy. After delivery, one of her glands became clogged, probably from the swelling that followed the birth. The opening to the gland was closed down and the gland itself became infected. When Pat and her husband had sexual intercourse, bacteria from the infected gland were being deposited into her urethra. The bacteria could then work their way into the bladder and cause infections.

A study called a *Tratner urethrogram* confirmed the diagnosis. We were able to demonstrate the track along which the bacteria moved from the gland into the urethra. Pat was treated in the office. I anesthetized the outer portion of her urethra where the gland opening can be seen. Then I opened the gland and let it drain. Within a few days, it healed naturally.

As proof this was Pat's problem, she never had another bladder infection. She has since delivered two more children.

Meredith is another patient with a similar story but who had a different problem. The mother of three children, she never had a bladder infection in her life until after the last child was born. Then she had chronic infections. She got them whether or not she had intercourse. Moreover, different organisms were cultured from her bladder each time.

Like Pat's, Meredith's uroflow and cystometrogram were normal. But her IVP—which reveals anatomic details of the urinary tract—showed a little pocket or pouch situated in the area of the urethra. A Tratner urethrogram then confirmed the presence of a urethral diverticulum.

After delivery, a small gland within Meredith's urethra had distended. Called a *diverticulum,* the sac was big enough to hold a stone (I actually saw this in one patient). Like a pouch or a mini-bladder, the diverticulum filled with urine. And the urine provided a stagnant breeding ground for bacteria. Meredith developed many infections as the bacteria migrated into her bladder. Each time an infection was eradicated, a new one, usually caused by a different organism, appeared.

Once Meredith's urethral diverticulum was surgically repaired, her infections stopped for good.

Sometimes women are born with diverticula. A very small number of women who have not had a child have this problem, but almost all diverticula appear in women who have had children.

* * *

Medicine in recent years has made great advances. Not long ago a woman with severe kidney disease could not bear children. Kidney transplant patients were sometimes even given a hysterectomy so they would not accidentally become pregnant.

Now, however, even transplant patients can have children because of improved management of pregnancy and kidney rejection. This was brought home to me when I was a resident in training at UCLA. During one month, I was apprenticed to the former chief of the department, a physician who had done pioneering work in kidney transplantation.

When I asked, "Can kidney transplant patients bear children?" he turned and looked at me, all the while chewing on his pipe. He then reached into his hip pocket and withdrew his wallet. I had absolutely no idea what he was up to. He took out a photograph that showed a woman, a man, and four children. He said with evident pride, "Look at this picture." I thought maybe it was his daughter and his grandchildren. Instead, to my surprise, this was one of his kidney transplant patients. After her operation, she had all those children—each named in part after the distinguished doctor. This photograph was a constant reminder to him of why urology is such a satisfying profession. It was a reminder to me of what medicine, at its best, can do to maintain and promote life.

NINE

Like Mother, Like Daughter: Safeguarding Your Child's Urologic Health

There are some agonizing moments in motherhood and one of them goes like this:

You put your two-year-old daughter on the toilet to urinate. Instantly, she puts her hand between her legs and starts to cry. You get that sudden clutch at the throat. She has been doing well in toilet training. Yet now she is in pain, saying her pee-pee hurts. It is almost impossible to get really useful information out of her. She's too young to tell you if it hurts when she urinates or after she urinates, if it hurts on the outside or inside. And she may be faking it, in an effort to escape the socialization of toilet training.

But there isn't any mother who doesn't panic when her child cries out in pain. It is not unusual for a mother to call my office at any hour of the day or night in great concern over the agony of her daughter's possible bladder infection.

Children are subject to the same laws of nature as adults. What gets in must get out. When, for any reason, bacteria are not flushed from the bladder in the normal course of urinating, an infection can ensue.

It is not normal for a child to have a bladder infection. The idea that it's "no big deal" to have three or four infections a year is as unacceptable in girls as it is for their mothers. Moreover, bladder infections in children should not be taken lightly. We are born with two kidneys that have to last a lifetime. If there is damage to these organs, a person must compensate for that damage for the rest of her life.

A few children suffer neurologic damage that results in urinary tract problems. Others are born with anatomic problems that affect the function of the urinary tract. Some defects are quite severe and get diagnosed early while others are mild and may go on for years before a physician detects the problem. Some are never picked up.

Most often, though, bladder infections in children are the result of a functional problem. That is, the urinary tract is not working properly even though all the parts are in the right place. With a little detective work, the cause can be tracked down and treated.

What would make you suspect your child has a urinary problem? She may complain that it hurts when she urinates. Or she may experience nausea, vomiting, and pain. Children with urinary dysfunction can have as many diverse symptoms as adults do. Usually, a child with a more serious problem becomes lethargic. She does not run around as usual, driving Mom crazy; she may sit quietly, hugging a favorite toy. Abdominal pain is a sign that something is wrong and you should take her to a pediatrician whenever such symptoms occur.

Amy

Amy's pediatrician diagnosed her as having a bladder infection. Since even one infection in a young child can be a sign of serious trouble, the doctor referred Amy to a urologist. If her anatomy was abnormal or there was a neurologic problem, this would be the time to pick it up. If not, at least her mother could rest assured.

At age two years and eleven months, Amy was one of those bright, determined little souls who could chatter your ear off. She flopped herself down in a chair in my office and began to swing her legs in the air. Amy's mother shushed her and then began to talk.

She poured out a great deal of emotion and very few facts. Since Amy was too young to give me facts, I had to rely on her mother for them.

I really wanted to know about Amy's voiding habits. Was she in the process of being toilet trained? Has she achieved nighttime control or does she wet her bed at night? How high was her fever? Was there blood in her urine? What happened in the twenty-four hours before her symptoms occurred? Does she ever come home from nursery school with wet pants? What foods does she like best? Is there a family history of urinary problems? Did Amy have any medical problems in the first year of her life? And so on.

Amy's mother said her daughter was completely toilet trained. She looked at her daughter and said, "Amy knows how to wipe from front to back, don't you?" The mother was quite adamant about this. She seemed to think that I was questioning her competency as a parent in asking how Amy was taught to wipe herself.

After the interview, I took Amy into the bathroom and asked her to urinate. She cheerfully cooperated. And as we chatted about nursery school, sure enough, she wiped herself back to front.

Because Amy so fiercely wanted to be independent, she decided she could manage her own toilet habits. Her mother had indeed told her how to wipe herself properly. And Amy steadfastly maintained—to Mommy—that she was following orders.

But alone with me, Amy admitted otherwise. She used the same piece of toilet tissue on her rectum and vagina, rubbing back to front. After all, she was her own boss. Like active youngsters everywhere, she was always in a hurry to get back outside to play. Amy would sit for hours with her friends and hold in urine so as not to give up the game or a toy. She even wet her pants at such times. This is a commonplace problem in nursery schools.

I explained to Amy that she was only hurting herself. She literally rubbed bacteria from her perineum into her urethra. By sitting on wet pants, the bacteria count to her urethra increased. The result: a painful bladder infection.

In assessing children's bladder infections, hygiene becomes extremely important. How many kids wash their hands after they urinate? As many of us note, the hand towels are always dry and the soap seems to last a long time in the kids' bathroom.

One way to orient children to the importance of hygiene is to follow what I did with my own daughter. She uses two pieces of paper, one to wipe from the front which is discarded into the toilet. A second piece is then used to wipe between the buttocks. She never uses the same piece of paper twice. This two-paper technique helps many children to get dry and stay clean at the same time.

Teach your little girl about her body. Use a mirror and don't be afraid to give her the correct words for her vagina and urethra.

Vaginitis is another problem in children related to hygiene. Even though children are not sexually active, vaginal secretions or urine on underpants can lead to urethritis and bladder infections.

Then there is the bubble bath syndrome. Chemicals in many bubble bath solutions will irritate the protective lining on a child's vagina and urethra creating a chemical burn. This irritated tissue no longer has a way to keep bacteria from adhering. Inflammation and infection may follow.

Foreign objects lodged in the vagina can also lead to vaginitis and recurrent bladder infections in young children. When a child has infections and no obvious cause can be found, she is often given a general anesthetic so that a cystoscopic examination can be done. The examination may include the vagina too. It is not possible to explore the vagina of young girls by any other means, and the cystoscope can take a look inside without traumatizing the child. You wouldn't believe what turns up. In naturally exploring their bodies, some young girls put pieces of toys, springs, chalk, or other foreign objects into their vaginas. This leads to recurrent vaginitis, which can promote chronic cystitis.

Pinworms are another hygiene issue. Young children playing in the dirt easily pick up bowel pinworms. You might notice that she has a scratchy bottom and seems to pick at herself. Careless wiping can spread pinworm infection from the perineum and give rise to chronic irritation of the urethra.

In terms of body hygiene, do not worry about repeating yourself if you think your daughter has not gotten the message. The effort you make is worthwhile. Good habits will last a lifetime.

Rebecca

At age eight going on nine, Rebecca was in the fourth grade at a new school. Like any new kid on the block, she was nervous. But for Rebecca, there was reason for extra apprehension. All her life, she had had the problem that she needed to urinate frequently. Sometimes at her old school she could make it to recess. Often she could not. In first, second, and third grades she probably had five to six accidents a week. These mortified her. Yet her parents told her she would one day outgrow the problem. She must try to control her bladder. If she tried harder, she could improve.

Of course, the worst happened. On the first day of class, ten minutes before recess, Rebecca knew she had to go. She raised her hand. The teacher did not respond. Then, to her shame, the boy next to her yelled, "Mrs. Smith! She has to go because she wet her pants!"

Rebecca's parents finally brought her to see a urologist. They knew something was wrong but had hoped it would pass. Rebecca did occasionally wet her bed at night but her main problem was with frequency during the daytime. The new teacher was the type who did not excuse children from class without a good reason. In her book, going to the bathroom frequently was not one of them.

My first step was to write a note to Rebecca's teacher. She needed to know that this student had bladder dysfunction. The second was to see, through questioning, if Rebecca might have severe emotional problems causing her frequency. In my experience, this is rare. Like Rebecca, most children with this problem are intelligent, emotionally stable children who happen to have true urinary problems.

So we hunted for facts. Rebecca told me that her symptoms of frequency often worsened after she came home from school in the afternoon. I asked her what she liked to eat. She said her favorite snacks were chocolate-covered bananas with nuts on top. And yogurt. Or cheese on toast.

As I made a list of the foods she liked best, it soon became clear that Rebecca ate many foods containing trytophan and tyramine. These amino acids promote the production of serotonin, a brain chemical that transmits along nerves found in the brain, heart, gut, and bladder. As described in Chapter Two, this nerve pathway responds to a limited number of neurotransmitters. Serotonin is one.

Rebecca's problem came into focus. She is a member of the teeny-weeny bladder club. Some children (and even some adults) have immature bladder membranes. They are born that way. In essence the final coating layer of their bladders has not fully developed. It is missing some components. This may be due to hormonal factors with a genetic basis. No one really knows as yet.

But the consequences are predictable. If you recall from Chapter Four, a normal bladder does not respond to small amounts of urine. The GAG layer is impervious to the charged ions in urine. But as the bladder expands, the GAG layer becomes less intact. A miniature leak of urinary ions crosses the GAG layer and tickles the nerves intermeshed below. This is the signal to void. It takes place only when a relatively high volume of urine is in the bladder, generating that tickle.

But a member of the teeny-weeny bladder club does not have a normal GAG layer. Her bladder does not have to expand to the same ratio to feel the signal to void. Indeed, relatively small amounts of urine are enough to stimulate the neural receptor systems telling them that it is time to void.

In treating Rebecca, I decided to first try some simple steps involving her diet. If changes in diet improve bladder function, drugs may not be needed, and as much as possible, I like to avoid medicating children. Some drugs have side effects such as dry mouth, dizziness, light-headedness, and even fainting.

The body breaks down certain foods and uses the products to make neurotransmitters. Some foods—chocolate, bananas, nuts, and yogurt—promote the synthesis of the neurotransmitter serotonin. (For a full list of these foods see Chapter Eleven.) Rebecca went on a low-tryptophan diet. With the by-products of this amino acid kept out of her urine, her symptoms improved. In just four days she experienced less frequency. Indeed, for some children, such dietary changes are enough to fully control urinary frequency.

When Rebecca came back to see me after one week on her new diet, she was better but still not comfortable with herself. She still could not "make it to recess" on some days and her goal was to last that long every day.

The second step was to give her a urodynamic workup. Did she have a neural problem? A normal uroflow shows a nice smooth curve as urine leaves the body. But Rebecca's uroflow indicated a high, quick voiding pattern. Her urine volume was small, but it left her body in a rapid, forceful manner. This indicated she had neurologic immaturity.

In this instance, children can be given an antispasmodic medication. The drug inhibits the response of the bladder muscle to neurotransmitters. The muscle is slowed down. It cannot contract nor respond as quickly as before.

Many times, a combination of diet and medication will be enough to prevent urinary frequency in members of the teeny-weeny bladder club. But each child must also be followed closely. After some time, she may need less medicine. Her dietary restrictions may be eased up. She may be able to tolerate a food once on the forbidden list. This same pattern can be seen in some interstitial cystitis patients; I suspect a subset of those patients have always been members of the club. Diet tends to improve their symptoms of frequency although they still experience the symptoms of burn and pressure.

When I saw Rebecca three years after her first visit, she was off medication but still watched her diet. And, she exclaimed, "I'm fine. I can make it to lunch nearly every day without having to go. And I haven't had an accident in a long time."

Prolonged Bed-wetting May Point to a Urologic Problem—And What to Do About It

Children with daytime urinary frequency may also be bed wetters. The scientific term for this problem is *enuresis*. It is defined as the involuntary passage of urine, usually occurring at night when the person is asleep. When bed-wetting continues after age five, parents often seek help.

Patty was eleven when she came to see me. She had been to other doctors and had tried different treatments. She never drank fluids in the four hours preceding bedtime. She slept on her back. Then on her stomach. She slept on a hard surface, with and without covers. Her parents bought a moisture-sensitive pad with a special buzzer that activated when she wet the bed.

But such interventions did not work. Patty continued to wet her bed, on average, three times a week. She did not dare spend the night at a friend's house. It was her deep dark secret; only her parents and her little brother knew.

In evaluating Patty, I first made sure that the obvious causes of bed-wetting had been ruled out. In checking over her medical records, I saw that complete urologic workups had been done on her in the past. There were no anatomic or neurologic explanations for her problems. If she had an anatomic problem, we could correct it with surgery; if she had a functional problem, we could treat it with medications. Her mind and body, however, were sound.

Patty's case, like those of many children, fell between the cracks. Her symptom of bed-wetting was real and, in a way, incapacitating. How to deal with it?

There are two theories now in vogue to help explain why children wet the bed. One postulates a sleep disorder and the other has to do with maturation of the bladder tissue itself.

Many children who wet at night are heavy sleepers. They do not wake up to the sense that they need to void. To help keep the sheets dry, many parents get up in the middle of the night to take their children to the bathroom. I remember my own mother doing this with me and my sisters and brothers.

Sleep occurs in cycles. During the night we follow a kind of roller coaster of sleep states. Stage one is light sleep that we can be easily aroused from. Stage four is the deepest, heaviest sleep, when our bodies are virtually paralyzed. Stages two and three are in between. During a night we move up and down through these stages. Dreaming occurs when rapid eye movement (REM) occurs.

Bed-wetting seems to arise in the oblivion of the first stage four sleep of the night. At this time, body movements and autonomic activity are intense. Nearly all children are difficult to rouse at this stage. It can take several minutes to arouse them to awareness, if they can be aroused at all.

It may be that some children are particularly heavy stage four sleepers, says the first theory about bed-wetting. That is, they are more affected by this deep, sedated state than others. They are even more difficult to arouse and awaken. And they do not respond to internal bodily signals such as the need to urinate when they are sleeping.

British urologist Mr. Richard Turner-Warwick has tried an interesting technique for bed wetters who are primarily heavy sleepers. He uses an egg timer. Each time the child has to void during the day, she must first turn over an egg timer and hold it until the grains of sand run out. She holds the timer longer each time until she builds up enough control to inhibit voiding for ten minutes.

Parents find that children tend to imagine that they turn the egg timer over unconsciously in their sleep, giving them enough time to come out of a deep sleep cycle and get to the bathroom. I have found this technique useful in getting children to awaken at night to go to the bathroom.

Recent research, related to what I have learned about cystitis, indicates the second theory—that some bed wetters may suffer from an immature urinary system. If the bladder's GAG layer is immature then certain neurotransmitters derived from food may trigger the bladder. The child wets without forewarning. Hence bed-wetting in some children is primarily physiological. They too are members of the teeny-weeny bladder club.

Fortunately, most children outgrow the problem. The sex hormones estrogen and testosterone affect components of the GAG layer. They aid in cellular maturation. With maturation, especially when the sex hormones begin to circulate around puberty, the GAG layer matures and bed-wetting disappears.

The reverse is true in older people. As discussed in Chapter Seven, when women lose estrogen they are prone to bladder infections, in part because their GAG layers become less mature. Immature cells do not make good GAG layers because loss of the GAG layer in the vagina allows more bacteria to latch on to tissue.

Bed wetters urinate frequently, perhaps fifteen or twenty times a day. But during the day, no one cares how often they go. At night, it matters because the sheets get wet. Many children in the club outgrow the problem at puberty when their systems mature.

Nevertheless, parents can get pretty desperate in the years between toilet training and puberty. Disciplines and rewards never seem to work.

One approach is to try various dietary restrictions, as I did with Rebecca. If your child has an immature bladder, certain foods would tend to exacerbate the problem. One of the major offenders is chocolate. It is high in the amino acid that is a precursor to the neurotransmitter serotonin. White chocolate, which contains no serotonin precursor, is okay. Children with enuresis probably should not eat corned beef, hard cheese, nuts, pineapple, raisins, bananas, or carbonated beverages. (See Chapter Eleven.) Restricting these foods for a while to see if it helps reduce bed-wetting is certainly worth a try to most families.

A few medications have been tried on bed wetters with some success. One is the antidepressant imipramine hydrochloride which seems to relieve symptoms of bladder spasm. The drug works by inhibiting the contractability of bladder muscle.

Another is the antidepressant imipramine hydrochloride, also known by the trademark Tofranil. It works by decreasing bladder tone—basic muscle response—and thereby increasing capacity. The bladder holds more with the hope the child can make it through the night. This drug inhibits another neurotransmitter, norepinephrine, that is responsible for muscle tone (the tension present in resting muscle) in the smooth muscle of the bladder. Ironically, antidepressants induce sleep. The child may be able to hold more urine but she may also fall into a deeper sleep and not be able to respond to her full bladder.

Given a choice, I prefer not to use antidepressant medications such as imipramine to treat bed-wetting children. The drug may compensate for the immaturity of bladder membranes by altering tone. But we can do the same thing for children by altering the foods they eat. (We can't, however, compensate for spasticity problems with diet.) Dietary and other environmental management help many children until their systems mature naturally and should be tried first.

In taking a close look at bed wetters, in fact, I found they have much in common with certain interstitial cystitis patients. Their urinary pH is alkaline and they show all the symptoms of a leaky cell membrane disease. I have treated children with the Gillespie cocktail (DMSO, steroid, and sodium bicarbonate) with the result that their bed-wetting stopped. These patients were only too happy to resign their membership in the teeny-weeny bladder club. This is a new and extremely effective treatment for bed wetters that is just now becoming known.

If you have a bed wetter, do not restrict his or her fluid intake all day long in hopes of keeping him or her drier. Less fluid means more concentrated urine, which might affect the chemical exchange gradients between urine and bladder tissue and might serve to make the bed-wetting more frequent. You may, however, restrict fluid intake in the two to three hours before bedtime.

Bed wetters, I would like to emphasize, do not have primary psychological problems. In fact, these children are usually very capable and bright. Bed-wetting is not, in my opinion, a sign of aggression, rebellion, or "getting back" at parents. These children do not need psychotherapists.

Desiree

Sometimes bed-wetting appears suddenly. Desiree was seven and had been dry (continent) for four and a half years. Then she began wetting her bed two to three times a week. Her mother was puzzled. Desiree was going through one of those stages in that she seemed very self-centered and demanding. Was this bed-wetting a sign of anger?

In my office, Desiree seemed like a normal kid. She did not report any symptoms of pain or burning but I suspected that she might have a low-grade bladder infection. A urine culture proved this hunch to be correct.

Some children develop urethritis without obvious symptoms. The bacteria get into their bladders but don't alter the surface enough for painful infection to occur. They experience—and usually ignore—some urethral irritation. During the day they may have to void more frequently but then they think nothing of it. Parents often do not notice.

Such urinary tract infections can first show up in children as bed-wetting. After years of total continence, they lose control at night. So if your daughter suddenly starts wetting the bed, she might have cystitis. Such infections, of course, can be treated with an antibiotic.

Other Problems That Undermine a Child's Well-being

Whenever urologists examine children, a primary concern is to find out if any anatomic defects are causing the child's symptoms. It is important to diagnose them as early as possible.

In some children, there is an obstruction at the ureteropelvic junction (UPJ), the place where the ureter enters the kidney. Called *hydronephrosis,* the defect causes the renal pelvis above the construction to balloon out from back pressure (see illustration). Urine still gets through the ureter but is greatly impeded. The renal pelvis then starts to hold urine in pools. It becomes a holding area for urine instead of a conduit for urine. The balance of the urinary tract is altered.

As a reservoir, the renal pelvis encounters the same problems of a bladder that does not empty. Pain and infection are not uncommon.

Hydronephrosis is dangerous because the increased pressure against kidney tissue can damage the kidney's glomeruli, the delicate little filtering units. The filtration mechanism may be thrown off balance, dumping protein into the urine. Permanent kidney damage can result. Hydronephrosis can be picked up with ultrasound devices even in utero, or it may not be picked up until the child is older. Sometimes the renal pelvis is as large as the child's own bladder.

The problem is corrected surgically. The doctor fashions a new uteropelvic junction or "funnel" so that urine drains properly, the idea being to ultimately save the kidney from damage.

Errors in the genetic code can lead to duplicated organs of the urinary tract. The most exotic in my experience was a man with six kidneys. Most duplications, however, involve a lesser degree of redundancy of the upper urinary tract. A common manifestation is multiple ureters (see illustration on page 218). Normally there are two ureters, one from each kidney. But there can be three or more ureters, all going to the bladder below. They can join together on one side anywhere along the tract and enter as

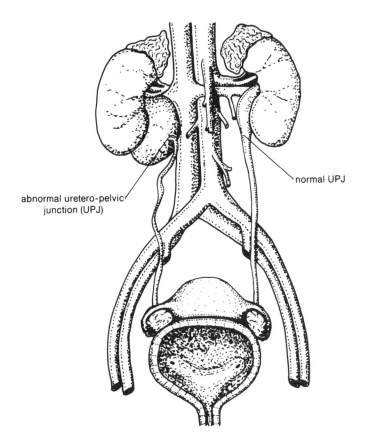

abnormal uretero-pelvic junction (UPJ)

normal UPJ

Figure 9-1, Swelling of the Right Kidney from an Obstruction of the UPJ

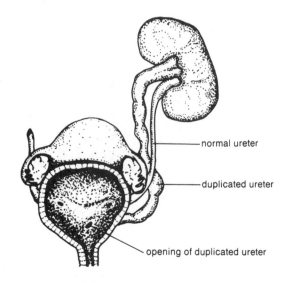

normal ureter

duplicated ureter

opening of duplicated ureter

Figure 9-2, Complete Duplication of the Left Ureter

one ureter. Or they can remain separate, creating multiple openings anywhere in the bladder or beyond.

A normal ureter enters the bladder at the muscular area called the trigone. The trigone has room for two ureters, one from each kidney. Extra ureters tend to enter the bladder elsewhere, away from the trigone. This creates problems. The trigone contracts when the bladder voids so that urine is prevented from flowing back up the ureters. But an abnormal ureter has no such stopper mechanism. Each time the bladder empties, urine may be forced back up into the kidney.

When an extra ureter empties beyond the bladder neck or into the urethra, the child will have wet underpants almost all the time. The tiny extra ureter drips urine all day and all night long. I once saw a twenty-three-year-old woman who continuously had damp underwear. No one had ever evaluated her problem. She did indeed have a duplicated system, with an extra ureter draining into her urethra.

But anytime urine is forced back into a kidney—a condition

called reflux—an infection is likely to occur. It can happen with multiple ureters or with the right number of parts. Infants with this disorder frequently have high fevers of unknown origin. The baby cries a lot and is called "fussy." Then when she is old enough to talk or at least point to the part of her body that hurts, the doctor may suspect an infection and take a urine culture.

Urine cultures of very young children are difficult to obtain. An adult or an older child can catch a urine sample in midstream, the best way to test whether or not bacteria are in voided urine. A young child, however, needs help to give a clean urine sample. Have her sit on the toilet with her legs spread wide apart. As she starts to urinate, put the cup underneath and catch a urine sample for her.

Refluxed urine washes back into the kidney like waves hitting the shore. And as waves erode the shore, the urine begins to erode delicate tissues that filter wastes from the body. If the problem goes undetected, serious kidney damage may result.

The problem of an abnormal ureter can be corrected surgically. It can be moved into a correct position and reshaped so that it closes when the bladder muscle contracts. The idea is to reconstruct what nature did not do right.

Much kidney damage in adults can be traced back to a presumed reflux problem in childhood. Some women recall having one or two kidney infections as children. But the problems cleared up. Children can have a mild amount of reflux that may affect only the lower part of the ureter. Such mild or low-grade reflux does not present a problem unless an infection develops and tends to disappear when girls reach puberty. Estrogen then affects the tone of the bladder base by thickening tissue. The ureter then closes completely and the reflux stops spontaneously. In fact, many children are not suspected of having reflux because it becomes obvious only if they develop a kidney infection. If they make it to puberty without an infection, the reflux is never diagnosed.

I mention these conditions as examples of what can go wrong anatomically with the upper urinary tract. As many ways as the body forms itself correctly, there are ways it can do so incorrectly. Fortunately, most of these conditions can be corrected with surgery.

No Strictures, Please

There is one anatomic malformation of the lower urinary tract that, while extremely rare, has caused much confusion in urology. It is called a Lyon's ring. Named after the French physician who discovered it, this congenital defect consists of a fibrous band of tissue in the urethra. When a girl who has this voids, her urethra takes on the characteristic shape of a spinning top. The urethra is essentially blocked by the fibrous tissue. Urine backs up and balloons the urethra. Reflux is a common complication. The Lyon's ring shows up clearly on X-rays and is not difficult to diagnose.

As a real stricture, the condition is corrected surgically. Under anesthesia, the urethra is dilated. The fibrous tissue is broken open and normal voiding follows.

Unfortunately, this rare condition has been used to justify urethral dilations in many children. When no cause can be found for recurrent urinary tract problems, physicians will sometimes dilate a child's urethra—that is, force it open with instruments— to "make urine flow more easily." The child is said to have a stricture in her urethra, even though there is no evidence of a Lyon's ring. As discussed in Chaper Four, strictures rarely exist in healthy women or in young children. External sphincters, a normal part of female anatomy, are mistaken for strictures. Urethral dilations are done on children as well as women, all because of misunderstanding of female anatomy.

As expressed in Chapter One, I feel very strongly that urethral dilation is a procedure *which rarely, if ever, should be performed*. In my practice I have only one patient who requires her urethra to be dilated and that is because, as a child, she had surgery done on her urethra that left internal scar tissue. She was not born with that scar, but today it interferes with her normal bladder function.

There is a handful of extremely rare neurologic conditions that can give rise to urethral spasms or other urinary tract problems. If your child is born with obvious birth defects, you need a urologist who is well trained in urodynamics to sort out the problems. *Urodynamics* is a relatively new field that examines the urinary tract as it functions, according to principles of fluid mechanics. You also need a good pediatric urologist. As has happened in most areas of medicine, urology is breaking up into subspecialties.

What's a Mother to Do?

If you little girl says it hurts when she urinates, there are things you can do to help her.

Have her drink lots of fluids. If the pain persists, don't wait more than a day to take her to a doctor for a urine culture. If she has a true infection, treatment should start as soon as possible.

If she has a high fever, you know she's really ill. If she's under two, you should use paracetamol instead of aspirin to reduce fever. Aspirin has been associated with Reye's syndrome, a fatal liver disease, in children and young adolescents.

Put her in a tub of tepid bathwater to bring down the fever. The lukewarm water will conduct heat out of her body. This is a good quick way to reduce high fevers in young children. Many parents are tempted to bundle up a child, thinking she will get chills. But to bring the fever down, you should leave her uncovered, with only a diaper, after taking her out of the tub. The air will continue to pull heat from her body.

If the child has to give a urine sample, be sure she does it correctly, as described in this chapter. Do not let her contaminate the urine sample, which would lead to the diagnosis of a bladder infection when none is present.

If she hurts and has no fever, try cutting back on bubble baths. Bubble bath does not carry infection. Rather, as noted, it alters the GAG layer and affects the way bacteria adhere to tissue.

For the child who has accidents but would rather play than go to the bathroom, you might try to develop a system that will reward her and make her responsible for keeping dry. You might give her stars or stickers each day that she stays dry. She should be aware of her bodily functions and how to control them.

Be on the lookout for yeast infections, which children do get, especially if they have been taking antibiotics for any condition. For children who have inborn metabolic disorders that prevent normal digestion of sugars, yeast infections are common.

Check for pinworms by looking for tiny white worms coming from the rectum or in the stool.

Even diaper rash can cause infections. If a child scratches

diaper rash, ammonium in urine affects sensitive tissue. A way to combat this problem is to dilute the urine by giving the child plenty of fluids.

Bear in mind that if a child complains of urinary pain and then runs out to play minutes later, the condition is not yet serious. Irritations usually resolve quickly, and children are very resilient little critters. But be sure they are not so stoic that they are hiding a serious problem from your attention.

A final word of advice. If your child has chronic fevers of unknown origin, ask your pediatrician to do a urine culture. If there is a problem with her urinary tract, the sooner you know, the better.

TEN

A Special Challenge: Facing the Changes Wrought by Cancer

If you have been diagnosed as having cancer, you should not let that overwhelm you. Your illness is something that you can cope with, given knowledge and support!

If you have cancer, you may feel angry, hurt, and sorrowful but you need not lose hope. There are certain strategies you can use to keep your spirit intact. And you have the power to make choices over which therapies to use, considering your lifestyle and what type of disease you have.

The Misunderstanding of Cure

When people are sick, they want to be cured of their diseases. But, in my opinion, medicine does not cure diseases. When we treat you for a disease, we might arrest its progress or alter its symptoms. We may extend your life expectancy. But every treatment for a disease involves trade-offs that can generate new sets of problems.

You need to discuss the many cancer therapies with your physician to find how they apply to you. Armed with information, you can make a conscious decision of how you want to proceed.

You can't make your cancer go away by thinking happy thoughts. A positive attitude will not cure you, but it will make a *tremendous* difference in how you live out the rest of your life.

This is an important point. When you are diagnosed as having cancer, no matter what the eventual outcome, you are forced to face up to your own mortality. Each of us has a life left to us, whether it be days, weeks, or years.

If you can accept the fact that one day you will die, you will begin to live.

Take a Week to React, Reflect, and Regroup

If you are diagnosed as having cancer, you should not discuss therapies and treatments right away. This is not a time when you are able to comprehend all the choices and make a decision.

No cancer grows so rapidly that you cannot delay a decision about what treatment to use. Instead you should take a week to psychologically orient yourself to the fact that you have cancer. You need time to go through several stages of coping with the information.

• The first stage is one of denial. You may feel isolated from everyone around you.

• The second stage is anger. You are furious, asking, "Why me?"

• The third step is to start bargaining. "Please, God," you may say, "if I do such and such, this problem will go away. I'll be good. I'll change, if only you make it go away."

• Fourth is a stage of depression. You may eat more or less, sleep more or less. It is a quiet time and a period of withdrawal. You feel helpless, thinking, "I'm now out of control. I can't take charge of my body."

• The fifth and last stage is acceptance. At this point, you may think to yourself, "Okay. I have cancer. That's it. I must deal with it as sensibly as possible."

*   *   *

These stages, drawn from research on death and dying by Elisabeth Kubler-Ross, apply to serious diseases such as cancer. You may not go through these stages in this exact order; you may feel anger before bargaining or depression before anger. In general, however, denial and isolation are the first feelings most people have after hearing the shocking news that they have cancer. And, given time, most come to accept the fact.

The best way to get through these stages is to let them happen naturally. If you are feeling temporary denial, it is not a time to have to face facts. Allow yourself to experience your full range of feelings. It will take more than a week to ten days to go through these emotional stages, of course, but the important thing is that you allow yourself that time to get the process started. You need to begin to feel those emotions and internalize the fact that you have cancer, before you go back to the doctor's office. This week is also a time to bring near and dear friends to your side.

Being told that you have cancer is like coming home one day to find that your whole family has disappeared. Imagine you find an empty house and are immediately faced with a plumber who says, "Ma'am, you have a broken faucet and I have to replumb the entire house. Tell me this instant whether or not you want me to go ahead." Being forced to make that kind of decision at that time is unfair. No one could handle it without time to prepare emotionally and mentally.

By the time you return to the doctor, you should be at the stage of having made a conscious decision not to roll into a ball and hide. You are taking one day at a time and concentrating your efforts on making each day worthwhile.

What Are My Options, Please?

When you go back to the doctor, about a week after you learn of your cancer, take someone to be another "set of ears" for what the doctor tells you. Someone who lives with you day in and day out might not be the best choice at this time; like you, he or she may be overcome by emotion. Rather, it should be someone who is not so emotionally involved with you that he or she would have trouble hearing what the doctor says. You need someone with you in that office visit who will say, "Right. What exactly are our choices here to help my friend?"

On this visit, the doctor will tell you what therapies or treatments are available for the type of cancer you have. Your laboratory tests will be complete and you have solid information to go on. Each therapy has something to offer different people. What you choose must be tailored to your needs—your age, the stage of your disease, your outlook on the rest of your life.

This is the critical time to find a physician who will allow you to be a partner in the decision-making process. Many people tend to worship physicians, thinking them to be somehow wiser than everybody else. How can I choose what treatment is best for me, I hear you saying, when I'm not trained in medicine? But you do know what's best for you. You can make intelligent choices. It is terribly important that you make an informed decision on what therapy to undergo. And then stick to it; don't look back once you've made a decision with a disease like this.

And please don't abdicate your responsibility in the matter. Some people let themselves be pushed into treatments. It is important that you have a physician who supports you wholeheartedly in your decisions, who will do for you what you want done.

Some physicians are not sensitive to individual needs. When one patient questioned her need for surgery, her surgeon said, "I'm sorry. There is nothing I can do to help you. Good-bye and good luck." He tried to make her feel guilty for wanting to try a nonsurgical approach.

If you do not like any of the choices offered to you, or if the doctor is pushing you in a direction you don't like, this is the time to seek a second opinion. You may want to hunt down an oncologist—a cancer specialist—who may be better versed in treatment choices. You should begin treatment as soon as possible, but only if you feel it is in your best interest.

In my own office, I discuss with patients the pros and cons of each treatment. I give them my opinion based on what I know about them as individuals, what makes sense to me. Then they decide if it makes sense to them. They choose. This way, I've never had a patient regret the way a tumor was handled.

Are You at Risk?

There are many kinds of cancers found in the urinary tract and I discuss some of the treatments now being used to combat them later in this chapter.

But who gets cancer, anyway? What are the risk factors in this disease?

Bladder cancer is the second most common malignancy of the combined genital and urinary tract. Only cancer of the prostate is more prevalent. In 1985 an estimated 40,000 new cases of bladder cancer were diagnosed. Approximately 10,800 people died. This cancer occurs most often after age fifty. Men are two to three times more prone to bladder cancer than women.

Bladder cancer is caused by many things. The disease affects people in every nation, but its rate of incidence varies from country to country, which makes us think that different environmental exposures are involved. People in Argentina are exposed to different chemicals, foods, and environments from people in Zaire, for example. As a result, their occurrence rates of bladder cancer are different.

As you can imagine, your bladder sees numerous toxic substances over a lifetime. It is a reservoir for temporarily storing the body's wastes, some of which are poisons. By and large, the bladder does an extraordinary job of removing these poisons from our systems without harm. Bladder tissue is fast growing and cells are continuously sloughed off in an attempt to rid the bladder of damage. Chances are good that you won't get bladder cancer.

But you certainly stack the odds against yourself if you smoke. Cigarette smokers develop bladder cancer two to five times more frequently than nonsmokers. The more you smoke, the greater your chances are of getting cancer. Cigarettes contain numerous potent carcinogens. When you inhale smoke, these poisons are filtered by your lungs and excreted into the bloodstream. The kidney then removes them and they pass in urine into your bladder. Cancer causing agents in cigarette smoke are known to favor the lung and bladder as sites in which to initiate disease.

According to toxicologist Bruce Ames of the University of California at Berkeley, a two-pack-a-day smoker, on average, takes eight years off his or her life. The amount of burned material inhaled from badly polluted city air, on the other hand, is relatively small. You would have to breathe smoggy Los Angeles air for one to two weeks to equal the soluble organic matter of particulates or mutagens (agents that cause healthy cells to mutate) from one cigarette. The air in the house of smokers is far more polluted and dangerous to everyone who lives there, than city air outside.

Other environmental carcinogens—things we breathe and eat over a lifetime—are also implicated with some kinds of bladder cancer. Common chemical cleaners (benzidine, naphthylamine, and 4-aminobiphenyl) induce bladder cancer in animals. People who handle these chemicals in factories are also more prone to develop bladder cancer than the general population.

People who work with leather, dye, rubber, printing industry chemicals, electric cable, paint, and metallurgic products have a higher risk of developing bladder cancer.

Recently, it was found that heavy use of phenacetin (found in the aspirin-phenacetin-caffeine compound called APC), once one of the nation's most popular over-the-counter painkillers used for menstrual cramps and migraine headaches, is linked to rare bladder cancers in young women. The research showed that young women with bladder cancer were seven times more likely than other women to have taken phenacetin at least a year before their disease was discovered. (Bladder cancer is most common in older men and rarely occurs in younger women.)

Heavy coffee drinking has been associated with cancer of the ovary, pancreas, and large bowel.

Artificial sweeteners such as cyclamates and saccharine have been associated with bladder cancers in animals. Although study results have not proven a link between such chemicals and cancer, you should probably ingest these substances in limited quantities. As with everything you eat and drink, moderation is the key to good health.

Many of these environmental agents are believed to be cofactors in bladder cancer. The theory holds that carcinogenesis (the rise of cancer) is a two-step process. In the first step, called *initiation,* something irreversibly alters the cell. The cell becomes abnormal or sensitized. The biochemistry of initiation is still a mystery. These changes remain unexpressed until the second

Stages of Bladder Tumor Growth

Bladder cancers are classified according to how deeply they penetrate the tissue. Each stage (see illustration) is associated with decreasing survival rates.

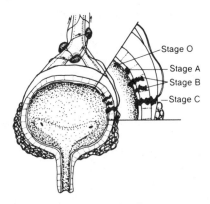

Figure 10-1, Stages of Bladder Cancer

• A stage O tumor is confined to the urothelium, the bladder lining. It only involves the cells of the top layer of the lining, just below the GAG layer, and it resembles a mossy carpet.

• A stage A tumor infiltrates other layers of urothelial cells down to (but not including) the bladder's superficial smooth muscle layer, the lamina propria. This layer contains a very thin muscle and should not be confused with the bladder's main muscle.

• A stage B tumor is one that has broken through the lamina propria and invaded the interstitium beneath. This is where capillaries and lymphatic cells reside and communicate with other parts of the body. Therefore, stage B tumors have the potential of traveling to other body sites.

• A stage C tumor invades deep muscle such as the detrusor.

• At stage D, the tumor extends to adjacent tissues such as the uterus, vagina, or lymph nodes. It may spread into more distant lymph nodes and distant sites in the body.

step, *promotion*—when a second agent, called a *promoter,* comes along to stimulate the abnormal cells into proliferating. Any number of agents in the environment called a carcinogen can cause initiation. But it takes a second influence, known as a co-carcinogen, to cause promotion.

Many suspected co-carcinogens, such as cyclamates, may be harmless when they encounter healthy tissue. But they can promote cancer in tissue that is previously sensitized, or initiated, by something else. Thus, even if we do not know the full story behind what causes cancer, we can as individuals limit our exposure to known cofactors in the disease. That's plain common sense.

Bladder cancer is insidious because generally there are no overt symptoms—no pain, no irritation—until the disease is well progressed. The most common early warning sign is blood in the urine. Since this is also a symptom of common cystitis, you should always get a urine culture done to determine if bacteria are present.

Women over fifty, particularly if they smoke, should get a yearly physical to check the early warning signs of bladder cancer. Some indications are bladder irritability, frequency, pain with voiding, or urgency. Sometimes lower abdominal pain and pain around the pubic bone are symptoms in later stages of bladder cancer.

Cancers of the urinary tract can be mild or severe. Some involve superficial lesions in the bladder that look like little fronds of seaweed. These *papillary cancers* can be surgically removed, sometimes in the doctor's office. Like warts, they may or may not recur. They involve what are called *transitional cells* on the bladder surface.

Most bladder cancers involve transitional cells. But about 12 percent involve two other cell types, *squamous cells* and *glandular cells*. Cancers involving these cells, squamous carcinoma and adenocarcinoma, tend to be more malignant and difficult to diagnose in their early stages.

Getting a Diagnosis

Because she is over fifty, June gets an annual checkup from her gynecologist. She has a family history of cancer and is prudent about seeing her doctor.

On one visit, June's doctor found minute amounts of blood in her urine. The blood could be seen only under a microscope but it was enough to wave a warning flag. June had nary a symptom of bladder distress. There was no pain, no frequency, nothing unusual to the eye about the appearance of her urine. With a lot of convincing, she agreed to see a urologist.

In my office, we proceeded to find out what might be wrong. I soon learned that June was a heavy smoker. This put her at risk for having true bladder cancer. But what type? Where was it located? What are all the possibilities?

First, June underwent an IVP. This test outlined her urinary tract so we could look for abnormal tissue. Sometimes a tumor will show up as an irregular shape inside the bladder. Irregular shapes in the renal pelvis or ureter could also be tumors. A dilated ureter could indicate a tumor outside the bladder that is obstructing the ureter.

Second, we ran June's urine through a cytology test. Since tumor cells are shed into urine, it is possible to inspect urine for abnormal cells. A cytologist looks at the first voided specimen obtained early morning and stains the cells. Abnormal nuclei containing different DNA can be noted by their unusual appearance. Some hospitals today use a special device called a *flow cytometer* that automatically identifies and counts tumor cells. Like an automated Pap test of the bladder, it is 98 percent accurate in detecting hard-to-find cancers.

Third, I looked inside June's bladder with the cystoscope. I was looking for papillary tumors, little growths that resemble warts. These are the most easily treated cancers and, indeed, June had one in her bladder. The size and location of tumors can often be determined through a cystoscope. If small, they can be removed in the office. If larger, they must be removed under anesthesia so that more tissue can be cleared away.

Treatments depend on how cancer is diagnosed and staged according to the classifications given in the accompanying box. There is no single definitive treatment that works against any particular cancer. A plethora of choices is available to you. Only you can decide what quality of life you want to maintain during any treatment.

Treatments for Superficial Bladder Tumors

June had a superficial stage A tumor, the type found in the mucous membrane and epithelial lining of the bladder. These tumors are unlike warts. Though not life-threatening at this stage, if left untreated they may become more invasive and gain access to the rest of the body, but like warts, these lesions can return again and again.

June's tumor was on a stalk but did not appear to have invaded more deeply into her bladder. I was able to snip it off, right in the office, by using a biopsy forcep or tweezer put through the cystoscope. The pathologist confirmed that she had a stage A, papillary transitional cell carcinoma. June then returned for periodic checkups—first every three months, then six months, and then yearly—for three years. If new tumors appeared, we could remove them before they had a chance to become invasive.

Superficial tumors recur in 50 to 70 percent of patients. There are many theories about why. Superficial bladder tumors may recur because a carcinogen has initiated changes in many cells, not just one. A carcinogen in the bladder would be likely to affect the entire lining. After all, the bladder is a reservoir for liquid toxins, and the carcinogen would bathe the bladder. Many sites would potentially undergo the two-step process of carcinogenesis. Or many cells would be initiated, waiting for a cofactor to come along and promote a new cancer.

Another theory holds that tumor cells slough off the tumor, float in the urine, and then "re-seed" at other sites, causing initiation of new cancer sites. It is one cancer showing up in multiple sites. For this reason, we biopsy what appears to be normal tissue in your bladder. That is, we take pieces of tissue from areas with no apparent tumor growth. Indeed, when other areas of the bladder are biopsied in patients, abnormal cells are frequently found under the microscope.

Maryann is also a heavy smoker who was found to have blood in her urine. She had several large wartlike tumors, which required general anesthesia and the removal of large amounts of tissue from her bladder in the hospital.

I find it odd that Maryann has continued to smoke heavily. For one year now she has had six new bladder tumors occur and removed. Fortunately, they were not invasive; they did not gain access to routes outside the bladder. It is her choice to continue smoking but she is willing to accept the responsibility for her addiction, which means more to her than her health. Although I strongly disapprove of her behavior, my role as a physician is to try to help patients as best I can. So I offered her another form of therapy to try to control, or slow down, the rate of her recurrences.

Chemotherapy—that is, giving drugs that kill cells—used topically in the bladder has been moderately successful in controlling the rate of recurrence of low-grade bladder tumors. The most popular drug is triethylenethiophosphoramide, also known as thiotepa. It is not used as a means of shrinking tumors that already exist; rather, its purpose is to slow down the process of recurrence. Since the drug is used directly on bladder tissue, side effects on the rest of the body are minimal. Some people respond well to changes in diet, cessation of smoking, and chemotherapy; they do not go on to develop more serious lesions. The drug is often given as a prophylactic, a guard against recurrence, after initial tumors are surgically removed.

Other drugs have been tried in patients with recurring tumors. Mitomycin C, instilled through a catheter to the bladder, has helped people who have frequent relapses despite surgery and other drugs. An agent called BCG (bacille Calmette-Guérin) is sometimes given to prevent new tumors. As of today, surgery is the only proven way to eliminate a lesion. Once the lesion is gone, the goal is to prevent early tumor cells elsewhere in the bladder from progressing into abnormal tissue.

Keep in mind that no single treatment has been found to work even 90 percent of the time. If there was one, everybody would use it.

Radiation therapy is rarely used to treat superficial tumors. It does not appear to prevent recurrences of tumors and is no more effective than surgical and drug treatments now available. But it has a significant benefit in a different stage of the disease, described next.

Treatment for Invasive Bladder Tumors

What happens to the patient whose tumor has spread to the interstitium and may soon be traveling through the blood circulation? A superficial tumor is like a carpet that can be taken up; an invasive tumor has gone through the floor and possibly broken up the foundation.

When tumors become invasive, the potential for a cure is greatly reduced. About one-third of patients who have bladder cancer show up in the doctor's office with invasive tumors. In other words, often by the time the symptoms prompt them to see a physician, their cancer is no longer superficial and may be severe. (Lung cancer is similar. The cancer is often advanced by the time the symptoms lead the patient to seek medical attention.)

If the tumor has broken into your bladder's communication center, which is the interstitium, you run a higher risk of your cancer going out of control. It may no longer be contained in the bladder. The deeper it is, the less chance that it can be handled by simply removing the cancer. At this point, chemotherapy is less effective. We have not yet found a medication or combination of drugs that will guarantee suppression of tumor cell growth.

However, there is hope. Over the years, urologists have been able to obtain the best cure rates for stage B and C tumors by totally removing the bladder. Called a *cystectomy,* the operation is done in hopes of removing the cancer before it spreads beyond the bladder to a significant degree.

Ruth sold real estate for twenty-five years and smoked as a way of appearing more businesslike. Five years ago her children got on her case and convinced her to stop smoking. Nevertheless last year she was diagnosed as having invasive bladder cancer. It appeared to be a stage B tumor that had broken through the lamina propria and into the interstitium.

A series of tests was performed to see if the cancer had spread. These included a CAT scan (see Appendix D) of the lymph nodes in her abdomen, a liver and spleen scan, and a bone scan. If the cancer had spread, those were the most likely sites it would turn up. Happily, all the results of these tests were negative. Ruth was otherwise healthy. This meant she had good odds of surviving the cancer if her bladder was removed.

Cystectomy involves removing the bladder, uterus, and ovaries. Because these organs are interconnected, they must all come out together. Once these organs are removed, the pathologist checks over all the lymph nodes removed with them. If the nodes are clear of cancer cells, the patient stands a good chance of surviving five years after her operation. If cancer has spread to the nodes, her odds are reduced.

In Ruth's case there was no evidence of tumor cells anywhere else in her body. Hers had been a true stage B tumor.

"I have a lot of living to do," Ruth told me. "I want to see my grandchildren grow up." Ruth took a very positive attitude about her situation. She knew she would have problems but planned to cope with them as they arrived.

Her first hurdle was to face the need for a urinary diversion. With her bladder removed, she needed a way to drain urine from her body. Various methods have been developed to divert urine and, as with other aspects of urology, surgeons differ in their approach of how to do it.

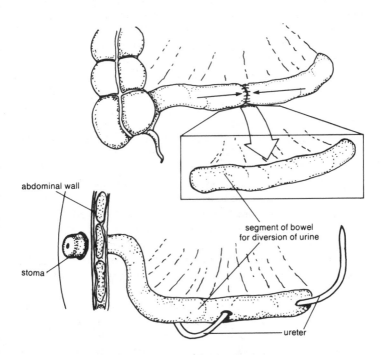

Figure 10-2, A Bricker Urinary Diversion

Most common is the Bricker urinary diversion. In this procedure, a small portion of bowel is disconnected from the stream of stool. Then the bowel is rejoined so that stool continues to come out at the rectum (see illustration on page 235).

This borrowed piece of bowel is then used as a conduit to get urine from the ureters to outside the body. It is simply a piece of "pipe" borrowed from another part of your body. The two ureters are attached to this piece of bowel, which is then brought out to the skin where it forms a stoma or opening on the skin. The stoma, which resembles a rosebudlike nipple, is placed below the waist. Urine drains passively from the hole and is collected in a small bag that serves as an external bladder. The bag is emptied as needed through a stopper.

Ruth chose this standard procedure over a newer one, the Koch pouch, a more recently available procedure in which a piece of bowel is fashioned into an internal reservoir—essentially a new mini-bladder. Instead of having a bag on the skin, a bag rests inside the abdominal cavity. A stoma is made through the skin, and to drain urine, the patient simply places a catheter through the hole and the urine comes out. With this relatively new technique, the urine is not collected outside the body. Long-term statistics on its advantages and disadvantages are not yet available. However, it is an alternative for those who have serious problems with body image.

As you know, outlook is important in coping with cancer and its aftermath. At her follow-up visit, Ruth laughingly explained that her urinary diversion had given her an unexpected benefit: "I can sit through an entire Dodger game, drinking all the beer I want. My friends all have to get up to go to the bathroom and they always seem to miss the home runs. I can outlast them all."

Some patients, however, balk at the idea of losing their bladders. Body image is paramount to them. In fact, I know of a woman who refused all arguments from her doctor that her bladder had to come out. To her, it was unthinkable. She said if that happened to her, she would never leave her house again. She would rather die than have a cystectomy and urinary diversion.

It is a physician's task to help every patient by taking her lifestyle into consideration. Like the woman who won't stop smoking, the woman who can't accept cystectomy must still be helped. Human beings have fallacies. Doctors need to work around them.

For this patient, the only alternative is radiation therapy alone. It is sometimes recommended to someone who cannot accept the loss of her body image. It may not be the best approach, but it was best for this woman. And it is better than doing nothing.

Proponents of radiation therapy point out that the five-year survival rates of their patients match those of patients who have their bladders surgically removed; others challenge these statistics. Your physician will advise you on choices of therapy and palliation. For example, an eighty-five-year-old with stage C bladder cancer is not a good risk for surgery; but radiation or another approach could provide some benefit. Each patient's needs and prognosis are different.

Urologists often combine radiation and surgery. The patient is irradiated to kill small tumor cells that may have spread beyond the bladder, then the bladder is surgically removed.

Chemotherapy is also used in conjunction with surgery. What if you are found to have a stage D tumor? Perhaps cancer cells have shown up in your lymph nodes but there are no tumor masses elsewhere in your body. This is when chemotherapy can be helpful. The physician may surgically "debulk" the tumor mass. Chemotherapy then has a better chance of killing tumor cells that have spread to other parts of the body.

Chemotherapeutic drugs are delivered via routes. They have different potentialities and affect different systems. No single agent of chemotherapy has been found to treat all aspects of metastatic (spreading) cancer.

One of the most successful drugs now used is cisplatin. It is delivered intravenously over a course of therapy lasting several weeks. Complete remission or shrinkage of invasive tumors is extremely rare when not coupled with cystectomy. But about a third of the patients treated with this drug partially respond. Another third find that their cancer is stabilized for six months.

If you have cancer, you need a specialist in urologic oncology. The field is changing rapidly and it is the expert who has access to the newest treatments.

Treating Cancers of the Ureter and Kidney

Cancerous tumors also occur in the upper portions of the urinary tract. They are less common and are usually picked up by an IVP exam. There is also a new instrument, the ureteroscope, that feeds into the ureters to view the interior directly.

When a cancerous lesion is found in a ureter, generally the ureter and the healthy kidney above it are removed. The remaining kidney takes over the job previously done by both kidneys. We cannot yet make a substitute ureter and calyx system, so the whole unit must come out. Also, cancers of the ureter tend to occur in multiple sites, so it seems prudent to remove the whole system, and the best cure rates are seen when this is done.

Unfortunately, cancer of one ureter can later crop up in the remaining ureter. Then the patient and physician are faced with a dilemma. You can't take out the only remaining kidney. The best approach is excising the lesions in the second ureter. The ureter can be hooked back up or a piece of bowel can be patched in to make up for the portion of the ureter that was lost.

Cancer can also strike the kidneys.

Vicky is a university professor of economics. She was healthy all her life. But on a routine physical, her gynecologist found blood in Vicky's urine. The physician did not waste any time. She ordered an IVP for Vicky and sent me the results.

Vicky had a kidney cancer, more properly called *renal cell carcinoma*. A massive lesion in her right kidney showed up on the IVP and was confirmed on a second test, called an *arteriogram*. The only cure we have at this time for this type of cancer is removal of the entire kidney.

This was the best course for Vicky. Her left kidney is healthy and is able to do all the work in filtering wastes from her bloodstream. There was no evidence that the tumor spread. For the past five years she has been fine and is back at work.

Vicky is followed closely, however, for such tumors can recur in the other kidney. As you can imagine, this has had an enormous emotional impact on her. She lives with the fear that a second tumor will grow as silently and asymptomatically as the first. It has not been easy for her to resume a normal life. As she said one day, "I've had to learn to accept my mortality. I don't take things for granted. I'm happy to be alive."

Exciting New Methods Promise Future Breakthroughs

Because our current methods have drawbacks, cancer researchers worldwide are looking at new ways to diagnose and treat bladder cancer.

One new treatment involves lasers. When I was trained, I learned to remove tumors using electrocautery. Today I remove them with a laser. The proponents of laser therapy believe it promotes less tissue damage and may be a factor in preventing the spread of tumors. We don't know if that is correct, but lasers are a new method of treatment that shows promise.

Conventional cystoscopes can easily miss certain lesions that could be cancerous. An experimental technique called *HPD* (hematoporphyrin derivative phototherapy) makes cancer cells "light up." HPD, a derivative of a natural pigment in blood, is injected into the patient and later concentrates in bladder cancer cells. When a cystoscope with ultraviolet light is inserted into the bladder, the areas with cancer cells stand out. The side effects of this treatment have not been fully evaluated and it is not widely available.

A whole new strategy for fighting disease using monoclonal antibodies will one day be tried against bladder cancer. Monoclonal antibodies are like "magic bullets," substances that selectively seek out and attach to cancer cells. If such bullets are attached to anticancer drugs, the drugs would be delivered only to cancer cells, and healthy cells would be unaffected. This would be a big improvement, since all of the cancer drugs used today kill healthy cells as well as cancerous ones.

In other studies, new ideas about carcinogenesis are suggesting new treatments. Damaged and dying cells sometimes release oxygen atoms that are extraordinarily reactive. Called *free radicals,* these atoms tend to damage cells with which they come into contact. Like meteors, they bombard healthy cells and knock through their protective surfaces. Free radicals are also introduced into the body by certain foods, tobacco smoke, air, and water. They are a part of the environment and may be co-carcinogens in some cancers.

However, there are ways to reduce free radicals in the human body. One involves taking in substances that are "traps" for free radicals. Their molecular configuration is such that it attracts free radicals and takes them out of action. Vitamin A compounds, known as *retinoids,* are effective free radical traps. Studies have shown that synthetic vitamin A inhibits cancer growth in animals. It is hoped such agents can be used to prevent cancer from recurring in people after initial treatment.

It will take a generation before we know if diet or vitamins can protect against cancer. The problem is, you are alive now; you can't wait for the final proof to come in. Also, we live in a world with numerous man-made carcinogens and co-carcinogens. It seems prudent to eat a healthy diet, taking into account the latest information on dietary factors in cancer.

You can maintain your body as you maintain other possessions. You repaint your home as it is exposed to weather, you put oil in your car, and you clean and repair appliances. Your diet is basic body maintenance. Just as well-cared-for property increases in value, your body will similarly benefit from proper care and nutrition. The next chapter is devoted to the important relationship between diet and urologic health.

Remember this common sense advice:

• Do not smoke.
• Eat a diet with plenty of fresh fruits and vegetables.
• Reduce your exposure to known carcinogens in the work place and elsewhere.
• Get regular checkups.

ELEVEN

The Right Diet Can Help

Nearly 100 years ago Thomas Edison made a prediction. "The doctor of the future will not give medicine," he said, "but will interest his patient in the care of the human frame, in diet and in the cause and prevention of disease."

The doctors of the future have not yet arrived in great number, but there are signs that Edison will prove correct. As never before, today's physicians are looking at the complex relationships between diet and disease. Dietary elements once thought inconsequential are turning out to be important factors in widespread ailments such as cancer and hardening of the arteries and in orphan diseases such as interstitial cystitis.

The problem is that most physicians are not well trained in nutrition. The subject is virtually ignored in medical schools. When I studied at UCLA there was not a single class on nutrition!

From the standpoint of urology, diet rarely has been considered important. But from the viewpoint of someone with bladder problems, diet can make the difference between a normal life and a life in constant pain.

Women with cystitis may notice that certain foods and beverages accentuate their symptoms of pain and burning. Alcohol and acid foods, for example, tend to increase discomfort. Men with nonspecific urethritis may feel better when they eliminate the very same foods that have been found to trouble women with interstitial cystitis.

It was these female patients, in fact, who prompted the first detailed look at how diet affects bladder function. They noticed that they could virtually turn their pain on or off by ingesting certain foods. Every time Janet drank orange juice, for example, she felt pronounced discomfort within twenty minutes.

An Old Wives' Tale Debunked

Unfortunately for many women, both with common cystitis and interstitial cystitis, the old wives' tale that says, "Drink cranberry juice to acidify your urine and combat cystitis," is just about the worst advice you could follow.

The rationale probably stems from the fact that women with cystitis tend to have alkaline urines, whereas normal urine is acid. Thus, drinking acid fluids such as cranberry juice presumably would make your urine more "normal" and less hospitable to any bacteria.

This makes about as much sense as putting out a fire with gasoline.

In actuality, the more you acidify your urine, the better bacteria like it. This is because bacteria use a component of acidic urine, called urea, to help them multiply and thrive. When the bacteria of common cystitis are present, they tend to make your urine more alkaline as they split molecules of urea in the process of multiplying. In other words, your alkaline urine is *the result* of a bacterial infection, not *the cause* of it.

When you acidify your urine in the course of a bacterial infection, you are helping the bacteria by giving them more fuel! And, of course, when you acidify your urine because your bladder is inflamed from interstitial cystitis, you fan the flames and increase burn to the tissue.

The Five-Minute Cystitis Checklist

But you can take immediate steps to help reduce your symptoms of pain and burning. For common cystitis, they are as follows:

1. Take one teaspoon of baking soda in water. This will alkalinize your urine and help deprive bacteria of what they need to grow. (Do not take more than one teaspoon, or you might suffer bowel problems.) One teaspoon of baking soda will work for about eight hours.

2. Drink lots of fluids over the next couple of hours. This will help rid your bladder of bacteria. The more you can void with efficient volumes of urine, the better.

3. Consult your doctor and *get a urine culture*. You need to know if bacteria are present to know whether an antibiotic will help rather than hurt you.

4. You can take the prescription-only analgesic Uromide, or the prescription drug Pyridium, to reduce pain.

5. Immediately eliminate all foods that have been found to bother interstitial cystitis patients (see list that follows). You do not want to do anything that might further irritate your bladder. When your infection has cleared up in a few days, after proper medical treatment, you may resume your normal diet.

The 24-Hour Interstitial Cystitis Checklist

If you have the symptoms of cystitis but no bacteria are found in your urine (or you have been diagnosed as having interstitial cystitis), you should do the following when symptoms flare up:

1. Take one teaspoon of baking soda in water. This will alkalinize your urine and help prevent the acids in urine from interacting with sore and damaged tissue. The action is rapid.

2. A few hours later, take four Tums or another form of calcium carbonate. Repeat the dose twelve hours later. This will slowly release bicarbonate into your bladder tissue.

3. Take the bladder analgesic Pyridium (available with a doctor's prescription) or Uromide (prescription only).

4. Drink lots of clear fluids. You want to dilute your urine. Remember concentrated urine contains more harmful elements that can interact with damaged tissue.

5. Experiment with ice packs or heating pads to see which helps best. Put those refreezable blue ice packs—or heat—be-

tween your legs, pressing the pad against your pubic bone and clitoris.

6. Avoid all foods on the lists below:

ACID FOODS TO BE AVOIDED

All alcoholic beverages, except for the wines listed later in this chapter
Apples
Apple Juice
Cantaloupes
Carbonated Drinks
Chilies/Spicy Foods
Citrus Fruits (lemons, limes, oranges, etc.)
Coffee
Cranberries
Grapes
Guava
Lemon Juice
Peaches
Pineapple
Plums
Strawberries
Tea
Tomatoes
Vinegar

FOODS HIGH IN TYROSINE, TYRAMINE, TRYPTOPHAN, ASPARTATE TO BE AVOIDED

Avocados
Bananas
Beer
Brewer's Yeast
Canned Figs
Champagne
Cheeses (hard and soft such as Brie, Camembert, and Tome)
Chicken Livers
Chocolate
Corned Beef
Cranberries
Fava Beans
Lima Beans
Mayonnaise
NutraSweet (aspartame)
Nuts
Onions
Pickled Herring
Pineapple
Prunes
Raisins
Rye Bread
Saccharine
Sour Cream
Soy Sauce
Wines, except for those listed later in this chapter
Yogurt
Vitamins buffered with aspartate

You will feel better in twenty-four hours if you follow the regimen just described. All six points must be observed for you to get relief and to control your symptoms.

When I first show this list to women diagnosed as having interstitial cystitis, most of them shake their heads in utter disbelief. Often these are the very foods they love and crave. "You don't seriously expect me to give up chocolate for the rest of my life?" exclaimed Stacey. "You've got to be kidding!"

I told her firmly, "It's your bladder. I can only advise you. But, like a diabetic, you can genuinely hurt yourself with certain foods. The decision is yours." Two weeks later, Stacey was back. "I was good for ten days," she said, "and then I cheated. I thought how could one little old avocado be harmful? Within twenty minutes my bladder started hurting. It was incredible. I knew oranges did that but never before associated avocados with the pain. What a surprise."

Mimi was hiking and, without thinking, ate a sandwich her friend had made. It contained aged cheese. "Within twenty minutes I felt pain," she said. "It took me a minute to figure out what had happened."

It is clear that if you have an attack of interstitial cystitis, you may have been exposed to or ingested something within the past twenty minutes that is likely to be the agent that promoted the attack. It may be the banana you ate or the chemical fumes you inhaled. In either case, you feel the intense discomfort of your bladder disease.

Since diet plays such a major role in interstitial cystitis, keep a detailed record of what you eat and how your bladder feels after each meal, if you think you have this disease.

Diet Matters!

Let's explore why the foods just listed can be harmful or irritating to sufferers of interstitial cystitis.

Two major groups of food are implicated in bladder pain. One is acid foods such as alcohol, citrus fruits, and carbonated drinks. They intensify a burning feeling in the bladders of patients. The other group is foods containing certain amino acids, the building blocks of proteins. Four amino acids are of particular interest to urology—tyrosine, tryptophan, tyromine, and aspartate.

As food ages, tyrosine (which is formed from phenylalanine) is converted into a special substance called tyramine. Foods high in tyramine are wine, cheese, yogurt, beer, and pickled herring—all to be avoided if you have interstitial cystitis.

Tyramine and tyrosine are problematic to damaged bladders because, once ingested, they help build the proteins called norepinephrine and serotonin. These substances are neurotransmitters, which means they carry messages in the brain as well as throughout the body. When these neurotransmitters are produced, a normal bladder feels nothing; the bladder membrane is competent and acts as an insulator. But the bladder of an interstitial cystitis patient is incompetent. It leaks. The neurotransmitters become active across the membrane and produce discomfort.

For example, if you have a bowel absorption problem and you eat foods high in the precursors to serotonin, excess metabolites may be excreted in urine. Again, in a normal bladder this has no effect. But in a bladder with surface damage, these by-products in the wrong spots can cause burning and swelling.

Appetite suppressants and diet pills work by raising the level of norepinephrine in your brain. The neurotransmitter dampens your appetite control centers. But the extra norepinephrine can torture the bladder of someone with interstitial cystitis.

Incidentally, when the brain levels of serotonin increase, you feel sleepy and calm. This may be why chocolate is the food of lovers. It contains high levels of the amino acid that helps make serotonin. When you are in pain or nervous, you may find that you crave foods that help produce serotonin, since it calms you down.

A second amino acid, tryptophan, is very often improperly metabolized by interstitial cystitis patients. An abnormal breakdown product of tryptophan ends up in their urine. As a charged molecule, it interacts with tissue to increase symptoms of cystitis. Thus these patients should avoid foods high in tryptophan, such as bananas, plums, pineapple, chocolate, and nuts.

The amino acid aspartate is found in meats and milk. It is also a major ingredient in NutraSweet, the trademark for the artificial sweetener aspartame. Aspartate is turned into phenylalanine—which is converted into serotonin, norepinephrine, and another neurotransmitter known as dopamine. Thus a high intake of NutraSweet causes extreme discomfort to damaged bladders.

How to Cope

Despite these problem foods, interstitial cystitis patients can eat a varied, delicious diet. All it takes is some imagination and willingness to experiment. Here are some guidelines to follow in making dietary substitutions:

• You may eat cooked onions in small quantities. Raw onions, on the other hand, are not allowed. Green onions are permissible, if you keep the amounts down. A tablespoon of onions will give flavor, whereas two cups of onions will cause pain.

• You can use alcohol or wines for flavoring. Just be sure to reduce the liquids through cooking so that the volatile elements in alcohol (the part that harms your bladder) are removed.

• You may eat a small amount of certain "forbidden fruits" if taken raw and in small amounts. One small apple or a half cup of strawberries should not cause a problem. But if you make apple pie using lots of lemon juice, you will have a problem because of the added citrus.

• You may substitute white chocolate or carob for chocolate in any recipe.

• Use the zest of orange or limes—that is, a little scraping of the peel—for flavor. Do not use the white part of the rind.

• You may use processed cheeses, such as American cheese, ricotta, cottage cheese, or cream cheese. These are not aged.

• Sugar substitutes can be a problem. NutraSweet contains aspartate, an amino acid that is related to the production of neurotransmitters. Saccharine contains elements that prevent the re-secretion of the protective layer on the bladder surface. Fructose, as found in Superose, is a safe sugar substitute and may be used freely.

• To make tea, dunk the bag in water only four times, quickly, just to color the water. By not steeping it, you will avoid tannic acid buildup. So-called sun tea is permissible. (Put three teabags into a gallon jar of cold water and let it sit in the sun for several hours.) Steeping in cold water reduces the acid content of the tea. Many herbal teas are fine for your bladder, provided they do not contain large amounts of citrus fruits.

• You may drink coffee that has had the acid removed. (Caffeine is not the problem for patients with interstitial cystitis, acid is.) Kava and Rombauts are two brands of no-acid coffee found in many grocery stores.

• You can buy a Toddy Maker, a coffee-making device, that uses cold water to extract coffee flavor from coffee beans without caffeine or acid. You merely add hot water to the homemade extract. Look for one in shops that specialize in coffee and tea.

• Wines? Many French sauternes and *late harvest* Johannisberg Riesling are okay. They have a high natural sugar content and a correspondingly low acid content. This occurs because the grapes are left on the vine until they overripen, and in some cases, turn to raisins. This special harvesting procedure produces a very rich and sweet but not cloying wine which may be served anytime—with dessert, with fish, or even alone. *Be sure to select only late harvest dessert wines.* Other dessert wines have a high acid content. Please note that all true sauternes wines are imported from Sauternes, France. Several American wines with the same or similar name are high in acid. Thus you should not drink so-called American sauternes. Visit a good liquor dealer to obtain or order the wines listed below.

These are examples of apparently bladder-proof vintages tested by my patients:

CALIFORNIA WINES

Chateau St. Jean Special Select Late Harvest Johannisberg Riesling, 1982

Joseph Phelps Vineyards Special Select Late Harvest Schreurebe

J. Lohr Late Harvest Johannisberg Riesling, 1981

Hop Kiln Winery Late Select Botrytis-Shriveled Berries Weihnachten Johannisberg Riesling, 1981

Hidden Cellars Botrytised Late Harvest Johannisberg Riesling, 1981

Austin Cellars Botrytis Sauvignon Blanc, 1982

Joseph Phelps Vineyard Selected Late Harvest Johannisberg Riesling, 1980

Alatera Vineyard Late Harvest Bunch Selected Johannisberg Riesling, 1980

Newlan Late Harvest Bunch Selected Johannisberg Riesling, 1981

Callaway Sweet Nancy Chenin Blanc Late Harvest with Botrytis Cinera, 1982

Freemark Abbey Edelwein Gold Sweet Johannisberg Riesling, 1981

Robert Mondavi Botrytis Sauvignon Blanc, 1981

Cakebread Cellars Rutherford Gold Sweet Sauvignon Blanc, 1982

FRENCH WINES

Barton and Guestier Sauternes, 1981
Chateau Bastor-Lamontagne Sauternes, 1981
Chateau Nairac Barsac Sauternes, 1980
Chateau Rieussec Premier Grand Cru Sauternes, 1978 and 1980
Chateau Couter A Barsac Premier Grand Cru Barsac, 1982
Chateau Climens Premier Cru Sauternes-Barsac, 1980
Chateau Luduraut Sauternes, 1976
Chateau D'Yquem, 1980

• You may drink carbonated beverages if you first get rid of the bubbles. Just sprinkle a little salt on your favorite nondiet soft drink and it will go flat.

• Home-grown tomatoes labeled as low acid may be used in virtually any amounts.

• You may freely use extracts (brandy, rum, etc.) for flavoring.

• Check the labels of drink mixes carefully to make sure citric acid is not present as a preservative.

• Imitation sour cream may be substituted for sour cream or *crème fraîche*.

• Pine nuts will not hurt your bladder. Use them instead of your other favorite nutmeats.

• You can make freezer jams and jellies without using lemon juice to set the pectin. This works with boysenberries, loganberries, and young berries.

Some patients, unfortunately, say to themselves, "Well, I just won't eat anything much. I can always stand to lose more weight." I strongly advise against that course. I have noticed that many interstitial cystitis patients develop the disease after going on repeated anorexic and bulimic swings. To lose just one more pound, they cut out foods that were beneficial for them and eventually altered their gastric and pancreatic function. The food they ate then was improperly digested, causing harmful elements to end up in their bladders and bowels. Indeed, I consider women who are anorexic and bulimic are women looking for another disease to happen to them.

A Diet for More than Interstitial Cystitis.

When I first began to prescribe these dietary restrictions, an interesting thing happened to many patients. Alexian, for example, had classic interstitial cystitis symptoms and was easily diagnosed. In addition to bladder pain, she had joint pains and terrible problems with her bowels. She complained, "If it isn't my bladder doing me in, it's my bowel. I can tell when everything falls apart. I get headaches and my joints ache." Having been to numerous doctors, Alexian was convinced that her headaches were psychological and that her associated symptoms were probably imagined.

Then she went on the diet. After the first week, she swept into my office as excited as a teenager. "I can't believe it!" she said. "My headaches are gone. I'm not bloated. My bowel movements are regular. I don't have leg cramps or hand spasms. This diet is fantastic. Talk about biofeedback!"

The next time Alexian came to my office she reported that her husband was also feeling better. His symptoms of prostatitis were completely gone. "He's even adapting his favorite recipes. He wouldn't dream of cheating on the diet."

Other patients said that when they cooked these recipes for the whole family, children with bed-wetting problems improved. Since many bed wetters have immature protective layers on their bladders, they do better when not exposed to certain foods that produce harmful elements in urine.

After a while, it became clear that these dietary restrictions were helpful to people with cystitis, migraines, nonspecific urethritis, early prostatitis, and enuresis. These disorders involve similar principles of how dietary factors affect cell membranes and neurotransmitter function. By following the same guidelines, patients of all ages and with very different backgrounds dramatically improved.

Intracellular Warfare

While putting patients on the diet, I began to prescribe vitamin supplements to make sure that each person received enough vitamins and minerals. Many taboo foods are extremely nutritious, and supplements can make up for what might be lost in following the restrictions.

Are supplements good for you? They may be better than you think. In looking at how diseases work at the cellular level, researchers in recent years have focused on a voracious type of molecule called the oxygen free radical. Free radicals are inherently unstable molecules. They have an odd number of electrons, which causes them to react savagely with other compounds. The ammonium ion in urine, for example, is a very potent free radical.

As free radicals roam through tissue, they bind to and change the structure of cell membranes, making them more permeable or "leaky." They can, for example, damage tiny air spaces so that lungs fill with fluid. In the bladder, free radicals can attack the protective layer and create leaks. This is the basic hypothesis for the cause of the disease we call interstitial cystitis.

Free radicals can be generated from food, tobacco smoke, air, and water. They are found in all biologic systems and may be a factor in aging.

Imagine, if you will, that your bladder lining is like one of those electronic bug zappers that kill insects on contact. Molecules in urine, in general, are like the bugs. They can't get past the zapper. But free radicals are different. They can explode the bug zapper and then allow other elements to get inside.

Fortunately, we can counteract these "superbugs" before they have a chance to penetrate the bladder's barrier through the intervention of antioxidants, which you get in your diet. Like scavengers, or little Venus flytraps, they envelop, gobble up, and inactivate free radicals.

What you eat and the supplements you take play an important part in this intracellular warfare. Many researchers think that if you are careful to take in adequate antioxidants you can help protect yourself against certain diseases. That is, you increase the number of Venus flytraps as opposed to the number of superbugs in your body.

The Natural "Poisons" in Foods

Many good foods, it turns out, are loaded with carcinogens, agents that may cause cancer in man and animals. If this surprises you, think for a moment about how plants in nature ward off bacteria, fungus, insects, and even animals. They contain natural pesticides or, if you will, poisons. Foods with built-in carcinogens are black pepper, celery, parsnips, figs, parsley, potatoes, coffee, cocoa, honey, fava beans, mustard, horseradish, cottonseed oil, and even that health food favorite alfalfa sprouts.

As surprising as it may seem, the dietary intake of nature's pesticides can be 10,000 times higher than the dietary intake of man-made pesticides.

What, then, is our risk of getting cancer from these foods? Haven't people eaten them for centuries and stayed healthy? Isn't anything safe?

Before you panic, rest assured that most of these plant toxins are not "new" to humans. We have been eating them for a long time, and we have developed protective mechanisms to defend ourselves against mutagens and carcinogens. For one thing, we continuously shed the surface layers of our skin, stomach, cornea, intestines, colon, and bladder.

We also have an impressive arsenal of enzymes that protect cells from oxidative damage. They are our built-in Venus flytraps. Furthermore, some protective factors are also found in foods. Several vitamins and minerals appear to be anticarcinogens. The most important antioxidants from the standpoint of urologic health are discussed below. I cannot, of course, give you precise dosages or recommendations on how much of any given supplement to take. Every person's biochemistry, lifestyle, environment, emotional state, and body weight are different. Thus I can only give a suggested range for supplements, with the caveat that you do not adopt a new supplementation program without the advice of your physician. Self-treatment can be harmful. For example, an excess of the supplement methionine can result in a higher risk of arteriosclerosis.

Medical Dietary Intervention Supplements

Vitamins, minerals, and amino acids work synergistically. You might think of your body as being a walking laboratory. The nutrients you put into the laboratory interact in extraordinarily complex ways—many of which are still poorly understood. However, research has shown that tyrosine works best with copper, vitamin C, vitamin B_6, magnesium, and manganese, while methionine, cystine, and cysteine require B_6, vitamin C, magnesium, B_{12}, and folate for optimal utilization by your body.

Interstitial cystitis patients should not take multi-B complex supplements: B_{12} is derived through a fermentation process; B_5 goes into the neurotransmitter cycle; and niacin is produced from tryptophan. The B complex in general works to increase serotonin, norepinephrine, and acetylcholine, which cause spasms, cramping, and burning. B_6 (also called pyridoxine), however, prevents undesirable degradation of excreted tryptophan in urine and is helpful to interstitial cystitis patients. Other antioxidants which are also of benefit include:

VITAMINS

Vitamin A

Helps protect vitamin C from oxidation.

As it is fat soluble, it can be stored in the liver. As all oil-based vitamins, it must be metabolized by the liver and should be eaten with food.

Suggested dosage up to 5,000 international units a day.

Betacarotene

Found in the yellow pigment in dark green and dark yellow vegetables (broccoli, spinach, cauliflower, squash, etc.) and deep-yellow fruits (nectarines, peaches, apricots, etc.).

Turns into an amazingly efficient quencher of singlet oxygen and other free radicals.

As it is water soluble, it is not stored in the liver, but can be stored elsewhere and should be taken in the morning and evening, either before meals or in between meals.

Suggested dosage up to 30,000 international units a day.

Vitamin B₆

This is the only B vitamin that interstitial cystitis patients should use to supplement their diet.

B₆ helps prevent tryptophan metabolites in urine from being used as free radicals. It may convert other amino acids into scavengers of free radicals.

As it is water soluble, excess is excreted in urine. Take it at night.

Suggested dosage should not exceed 50 to 100 milligrams a day.

Vitamin C

An important synergist in many nutrients.

Harmful for interstitial cystitis patients if taken as ascorbic acid and should be buffered with calcium carbonate. Calcium ascorbate is more easily absorbed. Vitamin C without calcium is like a gun without a trigger—you need both for maximum effectiveness.

It replenishes the calcium that is excreted in urine and helps store potassium ascorbate in cells.

It is a natural antihistamine.

Take in a corn-free base.

Water soluble. Divide daily dose into morning and evening.

Suggested dosage up to 2,000 milligrams a day as calcium ascorbate cobuffered with 500 milligrams a day of calcium carbonate.

Vitamin D

Helps calcium metabolism; aids in assimilation of vitamin A.

Fat soluble, so take with meals.

Suggested dosage up to 100 international units a day as cholecalciferol (vitamin D₃).

Vitamin E

Works to dilate blood vessels and helps prevent bladder spasms.

A natural antihistamine.

Helps absorb vitamin F. Prevents oxidation of fat compounds. Increases activity of vitamin A.

Fat soluble, stored in liver only for a short time, so take with meals.

Take in powder form instead of oil capsules (including oil of evening primrose). Oil capsules can go rancid, counteracting effectiveness of vitamin E as an antioxidant.

Suggested dosage 500 to 800 international units a day. (Doses over 800 milligrams can raise blood pressure.)

Vitamin F

Also known as EPA (eicosapentaenoic acid) and DHA (docosahexaenoic acid), a natural trigylceride marine lipid concentrate providing a dietary source of omega 3 fatty acid.

Makes calcium available to cells.

Is important for restoration of lipid membrane function.

Fat soluble; take with meals.

Suggested dosage up to 180 milligrams as EPA and 120 milligrams as DHA.

MINERALS

Calcium

It prevents buildup of toxic heavy metal such as lead and cadmium.

Important synergist for vitamin C.

Suggested dosage up to 500 milligrams twice a day.

Magnesium

This mineral is more soluble in urine than calcium is.

When increasing calcium, you should increase magnesium so as to help prevent stones.

Magnesium plays a role in the synergy between calcium and vitamin C.

Suggested dosage up to 1,000 milligrams twice a day.

Selenium

Like vitamin E, selenium is a potent antioxidant.

Protects the membrane of scavenger cells called macrophages.

Take as selenium dioxide (an inorganic form) rather than as the organic compound selenocystine or selenomethionine.

Suggested dosage 75 to 250 micrograms a day.

AMINO ACIDS

Cystine and Cysteine (levo)

These amino acids act as antioxidants and scavengers of free radicals. They are converted into one another with cystine as the stable form of cysteine.

Promotes healing from burns.

Stabilizes cellular membranes.

Promotes formation of carotene.

Involved in synergies with vitamins C and B_6.

Binds heavy metals such as mercury, cadmium, and copper.

Suggested dosage 60 to 180 milligrams a day.

Glutathione Peroxidase

Protects cell membranes from damage by free radicals.

Maintains integrity of membranes of red blood cells.

Assists white blood cells in destruction of bacteria.

Suggested dosage 40 to 120 milligrams a day

Methionine (levo)

A sulfur-containing antioxidant and free radical deactivator.

If you eat meat, you probably do not need to supplement methionine.

If you are a vegetarian, suggested maximum dosage is 25 milligrams a day.

PABA (para-aminobenzoic acid)

Important for utilization of protein.

Promotes wound healing.

Water soluble.

Suggested dosage from 30 to 100 milligrams a day.

Two other antioxidants are worth mentioning: taurine and dimethyl glycine. These are just being investigated for their possible inhibitory effect on neurotransmitters in the central nervous system. It is too early to recommend them as part of my medical intervention supplements, but they may ultimately prove to be beneficial for interstitial cystitis patients.

It is important to find supplements formulated without yeast, wheat, corn, soy, dairy products, salt, sugar, flavors, colors, starch, or preservatives. Look for the purest ingredients available.

When selecting dietary supplements, ask the manufacturer for its stabilization studies. How do they assure that the product lasts? Is there some type of moisture protection in the product? How pure are their compounds and what is their bioactivity? It is all too easy to buy supplements that are worthless due to poor manufacturing processes.

At the Women's Clinic for Interstitial Cystitis, I recommend "Cell Protect," a medical dietary intervention supplement. This supplement can be obtained through mail order only: The Women's Clinic for Interstitial Cystitis, 120 South Spalding Drive, Suite 210, Beverly Hills, CA, 90212.

It is gratifying to see interstitial cystitis patients who have found that they can hold urine longer and experience less burning, pain, and pressure while taking antioxidants. Antioxidants end up in your urine and help wage the war against interstitial cystitis and bladder cancer. When food is improperly digested, however, extra free radicals dump out in urine, causing a kind of "bubbling pot" reaction. The radicals release charges, which then result in leaky membranes and the flow of electrons in the bladder that are the "little electric shocks" felt by many patients. But when antioxidants are excreted in urine, they may prevent further damage to bladder tissue.

But How Do I Cook?

While vitamin and mineral supplements have helped patients feel better physically, dietary restrictions have shattered the self-confidence of many good cooks. As I have led women out of my office, they have turned and said things like, "My husband is Italian. How am I going to make pasta?" When I observed carefully and prepared my own family's meals, I began to realize how difficult it is to cook for a household when *only you* have a dietary problem. I saw that in every dish I prepared there was at least one, if not many, of the forbidden ingredients. Obviously, you need to be very creative to re-adapt cooking styles learned over a lifetime.

With that in mind, I called upon friends who are cookbook authors, restaurant chefs, and patients. We collected recipes that make it easier for women to follow dietary restrictions. These recipes have been collected into a cookbook called *My Body My Diet,* published by the Interstitial Cystitis Foundation. For information on how to order the cookbook, see Appendix B.

In bladder-proofing their favorite recipes, patients were helped in many ways. Of course, their families appreciate the tasty foods. But more important is the fact that women who take positive action in dealing with their disease are much happier and healthier than women who feel stymied and helpless. The knowledge that you are helping yourself is extremely therapeutic. The knowledge that you are helping others is ever rewarding.

Epilogue

A patient recently came to my office saying that all her bladder problems had recurred. The reason was quickly apparent. She had decided a week earlier that she simply did not like taking many pills. "I didn't want to be a pill druggy," she said. "So I stopped all my medications." She hung her head, waiting for me to say something, when she knew quite well what was wrong. Then she said, "Well, I guess every doctor's greatest difficulty is the noncompliant patient."

The story illustrates a quandary. For a doctor-patient relationship to work, both sides have to cooperate. The doctor's job is to educate, to advise, to counsel. The patient's job is to accept responsibility to tell the physician what works and what does not work.

The woman in my office was on an emotional seesaw. One part of her wanted to be well. The medications had stabilized her bladder for many months. But part of her thought, "Damn it all, my body should work after all this time. It should be well on its own without these pills." Within days of stopping her medication, she was right back into being a victim. She had abdicated responsibility for her own wellness. She wanted someone else to be responsible.

Unlike many physicians, I have no interest in power games of this sort. Instead I expect to relinquish control to you and merely serve as your adviser in helping you regain control of your urinary tract. But to give you this gift, you must listen to my advice, weigh it, and do what you think is right.

If, like the woman in my office, you choose not to take the required medications or follow my advice, it does not reflect on me. It is your choice. It is your body, your health. Only you can choose how you wish to live and manage your illness.

I use this story to illustrate an important theme of this book: Every woman should be an equal partner with her doctor. Medicine should not mystify and frighten you. It is mostly common sense!

It is possible to work with your physician in managing your health. But you cannot remain a victim. Victims are self-made. It is a self-defeating attitude that leads to fear and depression.

This book should convince you that knowledge and self-confidence are tools for forging a doctor-patient partnership. You now have the knowledge to avoid the victim mentality. But with this knowledge comes the responsibility to act sensibly. You certainly should not turn around and reject the medical profession because you think someone once hurt you. Urologic problems, as you have seen, are enormously complex. This book does not contain all the answers about urogynecologic disease. It is not a handbook for treating diseases at home. Rather it is a foundation that gives you an idea of how difficult and complicated these diseases are. It is a starting point for you to use in taking charge of your life. It should give you the knowledge base to use in finding an appropriate physician/partner.

You need to trust your physician and your physician needs to trust your observations. Medicine is an art, not a science. It is a continuously evolving process in which there are no edicts. If you don't tell your physician how you are responding to any given treatment, no one will. Without that feedback, your physician will not know how to help you.

I hope this book has met the three goals that I initially set out to achieve:

First, to teach you about your body. By knowing how it works, you can help assess how it goes awry.

Second, to convince you to take responsibility for your own health. You are a smart consumer of medical care as well as other goods and services.

Third, I hope that by giving you knowledge, I have given you power. If you use this power wisely, you will enjoy excellent health and well-being.

Appendices

APPENDIX A

The Interstitial Cystitis Foundation

The Interstitial Cystitis Foundation was established in 1984 to promote research into the field of interstitial cystitis and other women's urogynecologic diseases.*

This not-for-profit Foundation supports the psychological as well as the physiological needs of interstitial cystitis patients. It sponsors quarterly meetings for patients, with topics such as sex therapy, pain management, dietary restrictions, and mutual support. It publishes a quarterly newsletter for patients diagnosed at the Women's Clinic for Interstitial Cystitis in Los Angeles. It is the only newsletter in which all columnists fully understand the ramifications of this disease, as they are my patients. Regular features include a wine column, a self-help column (winning ideas need sharing), a cooking column, a psychologist's support column, and advice on sex therapy. The newsletter serves to keep all patients abreast of the latest developments in the treatment of this disease.

The Foundation also publishes a cookbook, *My Body My Diet,* which contains bladder-proof recipes by and for women and men with interstitial cystitis. Recipes also benefit people with colitis, migraines, and enuresis. If you are interested in obtaining a copy, please send your tax-deductible contribution of $20 to:

---

*The Interstitial Cystitis Foundation *is in no way* connected with the Interstitial Cystitis Association of America.

The Interstitial Cystitis Foundation
120 South Spalding Drive
Suite 210
Beverly Hills, CA 90212

Please allow six to eight weeks for delivery. Your donation will help support the Foundation, which conducts basic research on issues of cellular defects and their causes. Diseases under study include interstitial cystitis, bladder cancer, Epstein-Barr virus, abnormalities of the cervix in DES patients (daughters of mothers who took estrogen to prevent miscarriages), vascular tumors, diabetes, and inflammatory diseases in general.

The Foundation funds research protocols conducted under the auspices of the Food and Drug Administration. It is a national information resource on latest findings presented at urologic medical meetings throughout the world.

A brochure is available at the address given above. It describes the Foundation and up-to-date information about treatments used for interstitial cystitis and the Women's Clinic for Interstitial Cystitis in Los Angeles, where my patients are treated.

APPENDIX B

Pill Guide

What follows is a pill guide of commonly prescribed medications that affect the urinary system. It is not all-encompassing and it does not cover every brand name of medicine in a given category. Drugs are listed by types of medication, generic names, and by brand names. You will learn what each drug is, whether it is important to take it with food or without, its known interactions with other drugs, and what to expect it to do for you. In addition, medications that should not be taken by patients with interstitial cystitis are marked by an asterisk (*). These drugs will increase serotonin, norepinephrine, or epinephrine levels and cause pain.

This guide is intended to augment the information given by your doctor. It should not take the place of your physician in prescribing medicine. If you have any questions about a drug you are taking, call and discuss it with your physician. *Never* change medication you have been prescribed based solely on information in this pill guide. Remember: In order to maintain a working partnership with your doctor you must keep him or her informed of any side effects or possible drug interactions.

ANTIBIOTICS

Antibiotics are used to treat infections that may be caused by hundreds of microorganisms known as bacteria. A urine culture identifies the specific offending "bug" and determines which antibiotics will destroy the organism. This is called sensitivity testing.

In general, antibiotics are considered either bacteriocidal or bacteriostatic.

Bacteriocidal antibiotics kill the microorganisms they affect by interfering with natural processes in cellular growth, such as the development of the cell wall or normal chemical reactions. Examples of this type of antibiotic include penicillin, ampicillin, cephalexin, nystatin, and bacitracin.

Bacteriostatic antibiotics work by disturbing chemical processes (usually stages in protein production) required by the bacteria for their reproduction. Tetracycline, doxycycline, minocycline, and erythromycin are examples of bacteriostatic antibiotics.

Finally, there is a select group of urinary antiseptics which destroy bacteria by interfering with enzymes. Macrodantin and nitrofurantoin are examples of this category of bacteriocidal drugs.

THE PENICILLIN FAMILY

Generic Name
penicillin G, penicillin V, ampicillin, amoxicillin, dicloxacillin, cephalexin, cefaclor

Brand Name
Crystapen; Triplopen; Bicillin; Crystapen V; Aspin VK; V–Cil–K; Distaquaine; Stabilin; Amfipen; GX Ampicillin; Vidopen; Penbritin; Ampiclox; Magnapen; Amoxil; Augmentin; Keflex; Ceporex; Distaclor; Austrapen (Aust).

General Information
All the members of the penicillin family are manufactured in the laboratory by fermentation and by general chemical reactions and are therefore classified as semisynthetic antibiotics. These drugs work by affecting the cell wall of the invading bacteria. The medication should be taken on an empty stomach one to two hours after meals.

Cautions and Warnings
If you have a known history of allergy to penicillin you should avoid taking any of the drugs in this category, as they are chemically very similar. The most common allergic reaction is a

hivelike rash over the body with itching and redness. Occasionally there may be difficulty breathing. If so, discontinue the medication immediately and contact your physician.

Possible Side Effects
Stomach upset, nausea, vomiting, diarrhea, yeast infections, itching around the anus, fever, chills, changes in one or more components of blood, headache.

Drug Interactions
Aspirin or phenylbutazone will increase the level of free penicillin in the blood by making it more available to blood proteins. Probenecid will slow down the excretion rate in urine. The effectiveness of the penicillin family may be greatly reduced when taken with other oral antibiotics, such as tetracycline or erythromycin, which do not kill organisms but simply stop their growth.

Storage
Ampicillin and cefaclor *should be stored at room temperature,* while penicillin *should be refrigerated.*

THE SULPHA FAMILY

Generic Name
azosulfisoxazole, sulfamethizole, sulfamethoxazole, sulfisoxazole

Brand Name
Bactrim; Septrim; Gantrisin; Laratrim; GX Co-trimoxazole; Urolucosil (Aust); S–Methizole (Aust).

General Information
Sulpha drugs have several uses. Some are used as diuretics, others to treat high blood pressure or diabetes mellitus. As antibiotics, they are most useful in treating urinary tract infections.

Cautions and Warnings
Do not take sulpha based medications if you are allergic to them, salicylates (aspirinlike drugs), or similar agents, or if you have the

disease called porphyria. Do not take a drug in this family of medications if you are pregnant or nursing, as it will be passed to the child. If you have kidney disease, do not take this medication, as toxic levels may be produced due to lack of excretion by the damaged kidneys. Always take this medication with a large amount of water to prevent crystal formation in the kidney.

Possible Side Effects
Headache, itching, swelling around the eyes and soles of the feet, sensitivity to strong sunlight, stomach cramps, yellowing of the skin, arthritis-type pain, alterations in blood components, tiredness, dizziness, general feeling of ill health, sore throat, fever, unusual bruising, or bleeding.

Drug Interactions
When sulpha medication is taken with an anticoagulant (blood thinner), any drug used to treat diabetes, methotrexate (chemotherapy drug), phenylbutazone, salicylates (aspirinlike drugs), phenytoin, or probenecid, it causes unusually large amounts of these drugs to be released into the bloodstream and produces symptoms of overdosage. Avoid large doses of vitamin C, as the drug becomes less soluble in highly acidic urine. Also avoid large doses of para-aminobenzoic acid (PABA), as it as a competitive antagonist to sulphonamides.

THE TETRACYCLINE FAMILY

Generic Name
   *tetracycline, *demeclocycline, *doxycycline, *minocycline

Brand Name
   Achromycin; Economycin; Tetrabid; Tetrachel; Tetrex; Ledermycin; Doxatet; Doxylar; Nordox; Vibramycin; Minocin; Sustamycin; Deteclo; Mystectin; Ledermix; Austramycin (Aust).

General Information
   The tetracycline family works by interfering with the normal growth cycle of the invading bacteria, preventing them from reproducing and thus allowing the body's normal defense mechanisms to fight off infection.

Cautions and Warnings
   You should not use any member of the tetracycline family if

you are pregnant. Children under the age of eight should also avoid this family of medication, as it has been shown to produce serious discoloration in developing permanent teeth. It may also interfere with long bone development, resulting in retarded growth. Avoid this medication if you have liver disease. The tetracycline family may interfere with your body's normal sun-screening mechanism, causing severe sunburn. This family of medication should be avoided by patients with interstitial cystitis, as it affects the bladder. Do not take these medications after the expiration date, as the decomposing drug may cause serious kidney damage. Do not take these medications with milk, antacids, or dairy products, as they will cause inactivation of the medication. Doxycycline, however, may be taken with dairy products.

Possible Side Effects
Stomach upset, nausea, vomiting, diarrhea, rash, hairy tongue, irritation of the anal or vaginal region, anemia, possible brown spotting of the skin, fever, chills, and peeling of the skin.

Drug Interactions
The tetracycline family may interfere with the action of bacteriocidal agents such as the penicillin family. Do not take multivitamin products, which contain minerals, at the same time, as they will reduce the effectiveness of the antibiotics. Space them at least two hours apart.

Storage
The tetracycline family may be stored at room temperature.

ERYTHROMYCIN

Generic Name
*erythromycin

Brand Name
Arpimycin; Emsyin; Erycen; Erymax; Erythromid; Erythrolar; Erythroped; Ilosone; Ilotycin; Retcin; Erythrocin; Eryc (Aust); EMU–V (Aust); Ilocap (Aust).

General Information

Erythromycin is absorbed from the gastrointestinal tract but is deactivated by the acid content of the stomach. Because of this, the tablet form is coated in such a way as to bypass the stomach and dissolve in the intestine. It is effective against streptococcus, staphylococcus, and gonococcus.

Cautions and Warnings

Erythromycin is excreted primarily through the liver and should be used with caution by those with liver problems. This drug should be avoided by patients with interstitial cystitis, as it may interfere with the bladder.

Possible Side Effects

Nausea, vomiting, stomach cramps, hairy tongue, itching, irritation of the anal or vaginal areas, yellowing of the skin and eyes.

Drug Interactions

Erythromycin interferes with the excretion of theophylline from the body, resulting in toxic overdose.

NITROFURANTOIN

Generic Name

*nitrofurantoin

Brand Name

Macrodantin; Urantoin; Furadantin.

General Information

This medication is a urinary antiseptic which affects enzymes important to bacteria for growth. It may give your urine a brownish color, which is not dangerous.

Cautions and Warnings

Nitrofurantoin should be avoided by patients with interstitial cystitis, as it may interfere with the bladder. Do not take this medication if you have kidney disease or if you are pregnant or near term.

Possible Side Effects
Fever, chills, nausea, vomiting, rash, difficulty breathing, development of fluid in the lungs, arthritislike pains, jaundice, effects on the blood components, thinning of the hair, drowsiness, loss of appetite, stomach pain, and diarrhea.

ANTIDEPRESSANTS

Psychotropic drugs are used to alleviate anxiety. These medications affect brain chemicals called neurotransmitters, which cause such basic functions as sleep, wakefulness, and memory by altering the uptake of the transmitter at its receptor site. Each medication is designed to alter acetylcholine, norepinephrine, or serotonin uptake. As a result, some medications have anticholinergic side effects; that is, they prevent acetylcholine from being taken up at its receptor site. This causes the bladder to lose its ability to contract and empty efficiently, making it difficult to void. The tricyclic antidepressants are used by interstitial cystitis patients in low doses to prevent abnormal response to serotonin, a neurotransmitter which causes burning. Monoamine oxidase (MAO) inhibitors make you lose the ability to rapidly destroy tyramine in foods such as bananas, nuts, yogurt, wine, cheese, raisins, figs, soy sauce, chocolate, pineapple, and chicken livers, and as such should be avoided by patients with interstitial cystitis.

TRICYCLIC ANTIDEPRESSANTS

Generic Name
desipramine, amitriptyline, nortriptyline, imipramine, protriptyline

Brand Name
Pertofran; Domical; Elavil; Lentizol; Tryptizol; Allegron; Aventyl; Praminil; Tofranil; Concordin; GX Amitriptyline; Limbitrol; Triptafen; Motipress; Motival; Amitrip (Aust); Laroxyl (Aust); Saroten (Aust); Tryptanol (Aust); Nortrip (Aust); Imiprin (Aust).

General Information
These medications are effective in treating symptoms of depression and are useful in blocking the peptide-containing nerves in the interstitium of the bladder. These drugs are mild sedatives and may affect alterness. Appetite and sleep patterns may also be

improved. Imipramine has been used to treat nighttime bed-wetting in children but it does not produce long-lasting relief.

Cautions and Warnings
These medications should be taken with caution if you have a history of epilepsy, difficulty in initiating voiding, glaucoma, heart disease, or thyroid disease. These medications can interfere with tasks that require concentration, such as driving.

Possible Side Effects
Changes in blood pressure (both high and low), abnormal heart rates, confusion, anxiety, muscle spasms, dry mouth, blurred vision, sensitivity to sunlight, difficulty voiding, enlargement of the breast, increase or decrease in blood sugar.

Drug Interactions
Combination of monoamine oxidase inhibitors can cause high fevers, convulsions, and even death. These medications may interact with guanethidine, a drug used to treat high blood pressure. The effects of barbiturates, tranquilizers, alcohol, and other depressive drugs may be increased. Thyroid medication will be enhanced in the face of these drugs. Large doses of vitamin C *can reduce* the effect of these drugs, while bicarbonate of soda or acetazolamide *will increase* their effects.

ANTIHISTAMINES

Antihistamines block the effects of histamine, a naturally occurring chemical in the body, which is released into the bloodstream in response to a foreign, irritating element. This response is sometimes called an allergic response. Antihistamines can only block the release of histamine after histamine is in the bloodstream; they cannot prevent histamine from being released. Decongestants are often added to antihistamines in order to increase shrinkage of the tissue. Common decongestants include *ephedrine, phenylephrine, pseudoephedrine, and phenylpropanolamine*. Decongestants work by acting on the swollen vessels and tissues causing them to return to normal size by vasoconstriction. Decongestants should be avoided by patients with interstitial cystitis, as they will increase bladder pain by increasing the vasoconstriction already present.

ANTIHISTAMINES

Generic Name
chlorpheniramine maleate

Brand Name
Alunex; Piriton; Allergex (Aust).

Generic Name
cryproheptadine hydrochloride

Brand Name
Periactin

General Information
Antihistamines generally, and chlorpheniramine maleate speci-fically, act by blocking the release of the chemical substance histamine from the cell. Antihistamines work by drying up the secretions of the nose, throat, and eyes. Cryproheptadine works by competing for the serotonin and histamine receptors on a cell. This medication also has some antagonistic effect on the action of acetylcholine, a neurotransmitter.

Cautions and Warnings
These drugs should be used with extreme care if you have narrow angle glaucoma, stomach ulcers, or problems urinating. This medicine *should not* be used by people with asthma.

Possible Side Effects
Sensitivity to light, lowering of blood pressure, confusion, tingling of the hands and feet, blurred vision, nausea, vomiting, wheezing, nasal stuffiness. Use with care if you have a history of thyroid disease, high blood pressure, heart disease, glaucoma, or diabetes.

Drug Interactions
Chlorpheniramine maleate should not be taken with MAO inhibitors. Interaction with tranquilizers, sedatives, and sleeping

medication will increase the effect of these drugs. This medication will enhance the intoxicating effect of alcohol.

ANTIHISTAMINES WITH DECONGESTANTS

Brand Names
Actifed; Sudafed; Halin; Dimotame; and a number of others.

General Information
These products are marketed to help relieve the symptoms of congestion from the common cold, such as a runny nose, scratchy throat, or cough. These products are good only for the relief of symptoms and do not treat the underlying condition.

Cautions and Warnings
Do not use these medications if you are taking an MAO inhibitor, other antidepressants, or thyroid medication or if you have diabetes, interstitial cystitis, heart disease, glaucoma, or high blood pressure.

Possible Side Effects
Tension, anxiety, restlessness, inability to sleep, loss of appetite, sweating, nausea, constipation, drowsiness, difficulty voiding.

Drug Interactions
Do not take these medications with alcohol, tranquilizers, sleeping pills, thyroid medication, or antihypertensive medication such as reserpine and guanethidine. It is unwise to self-medicate with over-the-counter drugs in addition to these medications, as this may aggravate high blood pressure and thyroid disease.

AMPHETAMINES

Generic Name
phendimetrazine, phentermine hydrochloride, benzphetamine hydrochloride

Brand Name
Duromine; Ionamin.

General Information
These medications are used to aid in loss of appetite and therefore weight loss. These medications are addictive and highly abusable. They should not be used by patients with interstitial cystits, as they will increase bladder pain.

Cautions and Warnings
Do not use these medications if you have high blood pressure, thyroid disease, heart disease, glaucoma, or interstitial cystitis.

Possible Side Effects
Palpitations, dizziness, overstimulation, increased blood pressure, rapid heartbeat, hallucinations, loss of sex drive, constipation, diarrhea, dryness of the mouth.

Drug Interactions
Do not take these medications if you have taken an MAO inhibitor within the past two weeks. This may cause severe lowering of the blood pressure.

ANTISPASMODICS

Generic Name
propantheline bromide, oxybutynin chloride, flavoxate hydrochloride, isopropamide iodide

Brand Name
Pro-Bantine; Urispas; Stelabid.

General Information
These medications are prescribed for either bowel or bladder spasms. All drugs in this class will provide symptomatic relief only and will not treat the underlying condition. Each uses atropine or an atropinelike substance to prevent smooth muscle from contracting.

Cautions and Warnings
These medications should not be used if you have glaucoma, asthma, or obstructive diseases of the urinary or gastrointestinal tract. These medications reduce your ability to sweat and may cause heat exhaustion in hot climates.

Possible Side Effects
Difficulty in urinating, blurred vision, rapid heartbeat, nasal congestion, constipation, loss of taste, bloating, itching.

Drug Interactions
These medications may interact with antihistamines, phenothiazines, tranquilizers, antidepressants, or some narcotic painkillers. Antacids should not be taken together with oral dosages of these medications, as they will reduce the absorption. Do not use MAO inhibitors, as they may potentiate the effect of antispasmodics.

ASTHMA MEDICATIONS

Brand Name
Franol; Phensedyl; Tedral; Asmapax; Expansyl; C.A.M.

Ingredients
ephedrine, phenobarbital, theophyllinehydroxyzine hydrochloride

General Information
These medications are generally prescribed for patients with

asthma. These products contain drugs which relieve bronchial spasm, as well as a mild tranquilizer. Other medications in this class may contain similar ingredients which help to eliminate mucus from the respiratory passages. Any medications with ephedrine should be avoided by patients with interstitial cystitis.

Cautions and Warnings
Do not take these medications if you have severe kidney or liver disease.

Possible Side Effects
Shakiness, dizziness, dryness of the mouth, irregular heartbeat, difficulty in urination, stomach upset, diarrhea, chest pains, sweating.

Drug Interactions
These medications will increase the excretion of lithium. They will also neutralize the effect of propranolol. Erythromycin and similar antibiotics cause the body to hold theophylline, leading to possible side effects. Do not take these medications with alcohol or with MAO inhibitors.

MOTILITY STIMULATOR

Generic Name
bethanechol chloride

Brand Name
Mechothane; Myotonine Chloride; Urecholine (Aust).

General Information
These drugs stimulate smooth muscle and help to increase tone of the urinary and gastrointestinal tracts. By doing to they also help to restore rhythmic contractions and aid evacuation and emptying.

Cautions and Warnings
This medication should not be used if you have hyperthyroidism, peptic ulcer disease, asthma, Parkinson's disease, hypotension, coronary artery disease, or epilepsy.

Possible Side Effects
Sweating, flushing, cramping, diarrhea, nausea, asthmatic attacks, headache.

Drug Interactions
The effects of this medication will be negated by the use of any antispasmodics or antidepressants which have anticholinergic properties, such as Elavil.

URINARY DYES, ANTISEPTICS, AND ANALGESICS

Generic Name
phenazopyridine hydrochloride, methylene blue, methenamine hippurate, trimethoprim

Brand Name
Pyridium; Hiprex; Ipral; Monotrim; Syraprim; Tiempe; Trimogal; Trimopan; Unitrim; Methoprim (Aust); Alprim (Aust); Triprim (Aust).

General Information
The urinary dyes are often used as analgesics to help with symptomatic relief from a urinary tract infection. Usually they have little antiseptic activity. Pyridium turns urine an orange red colour; methylene blue turns it blue. Some preparations contain atropine or atropine-like substances to help stop smooth muscle spasms.

Cautions and Warnings
Do not take these medications if you have a folic acid deficiency, as this will cause changes in your blood. These medications do not treat the underlying problem. Do not operate machinery while taking these medications if they contain atropine or its analog.

Possible Side Effects
Itching, rash, muscle cramps, changes in blood components, nausea, fever, dry mouth, blurred vision, discoloration of the skin.

APPENDIX C

Tests and Procedures

CAT Scan

The CAT scan device gives physicians a "slice by slice" view of human anatomy. The technique (computerized axial tomography) is used in urology to view the interior of the abdomen. With it, physicians can spot cancerous tumors outside the bladder and view the kidneys, adrenal glands, blood vessels, and even stones in the ureters. A urologist might check a female patient with a CAT scan to see if any uterine or ovarian masses are affecting her urinary function.

Cystometrogram

This test measures the bladder's response to filling and voiding. Two catheters are placed in the bladder, one to carry water and one to measure pressures inside. (Some doctors use carbon dioxide rather than water.) The patient sits on a special toilet as a measured amount of water slowly fills the bladder. The pressure line measures the bladder's response to filling. The patient is asked to say when she first feels the urge to urinate. A normal bladder will be quarter full before the urge is noticed and the pressure gauge will show no response to filling. An abnormal bladder will begin to contract much earlier and the pressure gauge will show inappropriate response to filling. In this test, the bladder is then filled to capacity. When the patient must void, the water catheter is removed and the pressure line records bladder muscle contraction. In many such tests, the patient voids into a special instrument called a uroflow (see below). When a uroflow is measured with a cystometrogram, the physician has a good picture of how the bladder actually fills and empties.

Cystoscopy

This procedure allows urologists to view directly the inside of the bladder. The cystoscope is a long thin device with a series of lenses that refract light along a pathway. It is inserted into a bladder and the bladder is filled with water. Light shone through the instrument is refracted by water and is carried by the lenses back to the physician's eyes. Using cystoscopes, the urologist looks for anatomic abnormalities such as tumors or lesions in the bladder. Are the ureters in the right place? Is there stone debris? Other instruments to biopsy tissue or gain access to the ureters can be attached to the cystoscope.

Cytology

The cytology text is the Pap smear of urine. A patient collects the first urine of the day. Since it has sat in the bladder for at least six to eight hours, it tends to contain cells sloughed off from the urinary tract. The cytology test collects and stains cells taken from urine to look for abnormalities such as cancers of the urinary tract.

IVP (Intravenous Pyelogram)

This is an X-ray study that reveals anatomic features of the urinary tract. Special iodine is injected into the patient's vein, where it quickly travels to the kidneys and on down the urinary tract. The iodine is opaque to an X-ray device. The physician can view the outlines of the kidney, ureters, and bladder as the iodine moves along. The anatomy of the kidneys and ureters and the position of the bladder are assessed. Obstructions are located. Stones or tumors may be revealed. The test is purely anatomic; it says nothing about urinary function. (Note that people allergic to iodine cannot have this test done. If you are allergic to shellfish, you might be allergic to iodine.)

Lithotriptors

These are new devices aptly nicknamed "stone bangers." They remove stones safely and nonsurgically. The patient sits in a bath of water as the stone banger aims a special energy source onto stones. The stones break apart and small fragments soon pass painlessly from the body.

Tratner Urethrogram

This is the "double bubble" test in urology used to assess the urethra. A catheter with two balloons is placed inside the bladder. One balloon is inflated inside the bladder and the other is inflated at the opening of the urethra. Contrast material is injected through holes in the catheter. A special X-ray then reveals full anatomic detail of the urethra only. Diverticula, infected Skene's glands, tumors, or other abnormalities may be seen.

Ultrasound

This is sonar of the urinary tract. Sound waves are used to view anatomic features of tissue. The images are less clear than those of other methods but ultrasound is totally noninvasive and painless. It is safe for use in pregnant women and others at special risk for more invasive techniques. It uses no radiation.

Urinalysis

This is the type of urine test that can be done immediately in the physician's office. A urine sample is collected and screened for blood, pus, stones, pH, glucose, ketones, bile, specific gravity, and other factors. Bacteria are often found but can derive from pubic hair or other external sources. A urinalysis should not be used as an absolute test for cystitis. It is merely a screening test.

Urine Culture

A urine culture is the definitive test for bacterial infection of the urinary tract. The patient must take great care to collect urine voided in midstream to avoid contamination with external bacteria. The sample is cultured for twenty-four hours on special growth media. The type and extent of bacterial infection can then be determined.

Uroflow

This test measures the patient's flow rate. She sits on a special toilet seat and voids with a full bladder. The weight and duration of urinary flow moves an arm on a special graphing device below. This measures the speed and rate at which she voids.

Voiding Cystourethrogram (VCUG)

This is an X-ray study done to determine the anatomic position of the bladder neck and to check the position of the ureters to assess reflux (the backward flow of urine.) A catheter is placed in the bladder and contrast material is added. The X-ray shows the angle of support to the bladder neck and to the base of the bladder. The catheter is removed and the patient is asked to cough or strain. If urine leaks out, the condition known as stress incontinence can be diagnosed. Urinary stress incontinence results from a lack of support which prevents the bladder neck from closing strongly enough to keep urine from passing when you suddenly cough, sneeze, or laugh. If the contrast material goes up toward the kidneys, the patient is shown to have reflux.

Index